Basic Methods for Mental Health Practitioners

Basic Methods for Mental Health Practitioners

Marvin W. Kahn
University of Arizona

Winthrop Publishers, Inc.
Cambridge, Massachusetts

ISBN 0-87626-052-0

Cover Design by Janis Capone
Interior Design by Sharon Glassman
Copyediting and Production by Raeia Maes
Text Composition in VIP Palatino by DEKR Corporation

10 9 8 7 6 5 4 3 2 1

*To the Papago Indians, the Townsville
Australia Aborigines and Islanders, and to the
idea of mental health services conceived,
controlled, and provided by the indigenous
people concerned.*

CONTENTS

Know yourself

3

How people get that way: Coping and adjusting to stress and frustration

4

Recognizing the signs and types of emotional disorder

5

Clinical Methods and Techniques *Part* **II**

Clinical interviewing

6

Crisis treatment and suicide prevention: Intervention and therapy

7

Marital and family treatment methods

8

Problem drinking and alcoholism: Effects and treatment

9

Special intervention methods briefly

10

Prevention and evaluation

11

PREFACE

The intent of this book is to provide a basic orientation and foundation in the concepts needed, and in the skills required, by those who provide mental health services to others.

Many disciplines engage in providing such services. The range of training and education involved is extreme to say the least. It goes from doctorate level training for psychologists and psychiatrists to "learn as you do" in some paraprofessional programs. What is covered here is what we consider more or less fundamental and common to all levels in this diverse field. It is intended as a basic introduction to the fundamentals for those who may go on to more technical and professional education in this field and as a basic core of understanding and of methods for the paraprofessional workers who will have immediate need in applications for carrying out their work.

The book has grown out of the author's experience over almost ten years in developing community mental health programs by and for socioeconomically impoverished groups. The emphasis in these programs has been to develop the indigenous paraprofessionals' ability to provide mental health services for their own people in their own community settings. The kinds of information and the types of clinical skills that these paraprofessionals needed in order to be effective in their communities emerged from the experience with those programs. Since there was no satisfactory single source of training materials for this purpose, the need for a book such as this was obvious. The fact that many paraprofessionals receive little if any formal training is apparently partly a result of a dearth of appropriate training materials.

Some of what is covered here is treated at a much more elaborate, detailed, and higher level in many advanced texts. What is different in this book is the manner in which the areas and skills covered are put together so as to provide fundamental background and basic techniques that are practicable in areas where mental health workers are most likely to meet problems, without an approach that is overwhelmingly technical or too complex for comprehension by those without substantial prior technical education. Yet we have tried to avoid talking down to the reader. For these reasons, we consider it a reasonable basic introduction for both the journeyman level of those who have need for relatively immediate and direct applications and as an introductory step for those who may be considering or planning to go on to a more technical and professional education in this field.

While this training approach was developed for groups from very unique cultures, the Papago Indian tribe in the United States and an urban community of Aborigines in Australia, it is not written from a standpoint of either of these unique cultures. Rather, the basics and the principles are presented more or less from the standpoint from which they were developed, generally for white, middleclass, industrialized society. What our experience has shown is that these methods are basic and effective when they are adapted to the particular cultural group for whom they are to be used. What is contained here is a rather generalized form of the material. To be most useful the material must be considered in terms of the target group. This requires consideration of how each topic fits with the expectations, values, and customs of the group to which it will be applied. The trainees themselves, to the extent that they are representatives of the people whom they are going to serve, are excellent criteria for helping to put these methods into the proper cultural perspective.

— *M. W. K.*
university of arizona

Basic Methods for Mental Health Practitioners

Part I

Fundamental Concepts Briefly

While the emphasis of this book is on the methods, techniques, and skills used in mental health work, the effective and proper use of those methods, techniques, and skills depends on adequate knowledge of the basic concepts that underlie mental health intervention.

Part 1 is a very brief, condensed presentation of the major background areas. For those who have had previous courses in these foundation areas, it should provide a review and refresher experience. For those who have not had formal or detailed background in these fundamental areas, it is intended as an introduction and orientation. It is not intended as a substitute for the thorough and detailed consideration of these areas. Rather, for those new to this field, it is intended as a first consideration of what will need to be studied in much more breadth and depth in order to become fully and effectively proficient in mental health methods.

The field of mental health: What mental health work is all about

Mental health is concerned with helping people

Mental health is concerned with people. It is concerned with helping people who are having difficulty in adjusting and getting along with their families, with their friends, at their job, or in their communities. It is also concerned with people who are tormented within themselves, be it feeling tense, jumpy, or irritable; depressed, sad, or unhappy; feeling angry, mean, suspicious, or untrusting. Further, it is concerned with those who cannot control their drinking or intake of other drugs and with those who repeatedly get into trouble with the law.

Mental health also refers to concern with the factors that cause people to be poorly adjusted in their life situations or to feel internally miserable, as well as with concern for preventing such disorders. This latter is a task of mental health which is of equal importance to that of helping those who are already having the difficulties. For instance, if we know that children who are wanted, loved, and well cared for are likely to grow up to be emotionally healthy, stable adults and that those who are unwanted, ill-treated, and neglected are likely to have major emotional difficulties, then preventive efforts within the family before the problems arise would be important. If people drink more and if families break up more when there are no jobs, then prevention of emotional disorders lies not just in the family but also in the economic and social conditions of the community. Preventive measures to ensure mental health must be concerned with social and economic conditions as well as individual and family matters.

An example of one of the many kinds of mental health problems is the case of Angela. Angela was a sixteen-year-old high school student. She was the second oldest of six children. Her mother had health problems and a drinking problem. Angela had to do much of the housework and had to provide much of the care for her younger brothers and sisters. She had never known her real father. Various men lived with her mother for periods of time, but they seldom stayed very long. The family's income was from various government welfare programs.

In school Angela was a poor uninterested student. She dressed shabbily and had no real friends. She was frequently absent. When she was at school, Angela was very quiet, stayed by herself, and seemed shy and frightened.

One morning at school a student saw blood on the floor near a toilet. She told a teacher, who discovered Angela sitting on the toilet holding her wrists, which she had cut deeply in a suicide attempt. Angela was taken to a hospital and recovered. It was found out that she had been deeply depressed over her home situation for a long time. The decision to kill herself came after her mother's latest boyfriend had forced her to have sex relations.

Angela was entered into mental health treatment for her depression and for her suicidal inclinations. Her home situation was investigated and she was placed in a foster home, while continuing her mental health treatment. Angela's mother was also brought in to treatment for her drinking and for many other problems. The mother was allowed to keep the other children, but the situation at home was closely watched by child protection agencies. The man who raped Angela disappeared and could not be found by the police.

Is mental illness really an illness?

Although we generally talk about mental health and mental illness as if it were a sickness like physical disorders such as measles or a broken arm, it is clear that much of mental illness is not quite the same as most physical illnesses. There are some mental illnesses that are associated with disease or damage to the body, but most of what is called mental illness is not. Many people today argue that such conditions are better called problems in living rather than illness because in order to have an illness something must be found wrong with the body.

They also argue that calling such problems illness comes from times when such conditions were considered to be caused by the devil or bad spirits or by deliberate bad intentions on the part of the person having the disorder. In earlier times, considering such behavior the result of illness protected such people from severe punishments given those thought to be possessed and it put an emphasis on treating them. Those who favor the problems in living concept argue that it is no longer necessary to protect disturbed individuals by calling their disorders an illness. Furthermore, they see the disadvantage to the illness model being that the person is considered not responsible for his or her own behavior because what the person does is caused by the sickness.

But most people still regard emotional disturbance as an illness. Even though there is no physical disease and damage, they nevertheless feel that if the person isn't functioning adequately, it is not deliberate behavior on the part of the disturbed person but that it is due to the person's response to threat and stress over which the person may have little or no control.

There are a few, however, who are even more extreme and feel that all such behavioral maladjustments really do have a physical cause even if it hasn't been discovered yet and look to physical treatments and medicines for the cure.

For many practical purposes right now it matters little whether we call what we are dealing with illness or problems in living. In most cases, the methods and techniques we use will be the same. These will largely be psychological means of helping individuals to relieve their uncomfortable feelings, to understand their behavior and actions better, to accept themselves more fully and to be able to make changes in the way they do things, look at things, and feel about things.

Normal and abnormal behavior

There is no one ideal type of behavior that is normal. Rather, there is a wide range of behaviors that can be quite different and yet be considered normal. Furthermore, there is no sharp dividing line between what is considered normal and what is considered abnormal. Often it depends on the situation and the cultural setting.

Statistical cultural deviance definition

There are several main ways in which normality and abnormality can be viewed. One is in terms of the extent to which behavior deviates or is different from the usual behavior of a particular culture or social group. The more unusual the behavior is for that group, the more likely it is to be thought of as abnormal.

For instance, in modern Western society it would be very unusual for a person to hear voices that no one else heard telling them that they had been chosen to do the work of the Lord. But such an experience might not be considered unusual or strange in another cultural group with certain religious beliefs. When deciding whether or not a given behavior is normal or not, it is very important to consider what the cultural reference point is for the person who has had the strange experience or behavior.

Symptom definition

A second way of looking at abnormality or normality has to do with the extent to which someone has or does not have the symptoms of the classical types of mental illness. Thus, freedom from such symptoms as severe anxiety, depression, compulsions, delusions, or antisocial acts would suggest normality and having any of these symptoms would suggest abnormality.

Internal suffering definition

Some people show to others little of the turmoil and distress they are feeling. They may manage to continue to do what they have to in order to function, but they suffer greatly within themselves from feelings of anxiety, depression, or doubt. Such internal feelings also may be considered symptoms of mental illness, even though they are really only known through the report of the affected person. Extreme internal distress for a long period of time does deviate from the experience of most people within the culture, and simply by its unusualness it could be considered abnormal from that point of view as well.

Realistic problem solving definition

Another way of looking at this is more from the standpoint of how one regards oneself and deals with problems. In this point of view being realistic about oneself and one's situations, knowing oneself and accepting oneself, working toward one's goals and ambitions through having developed good problem-solving methods for living would be considered an effective, well-adjusted person.

Maximizing potential definition

Still another standard for normality is that of maximizing one's potential. The closer one can come to achieving full use of one's potential capacities in all areas, the closer one would be considered to have reached an ideal adjustment.

It should be clear that people exist in a world full of stresses and problems. Being and remaining emotionally healthy involves constantly meeting, coping with, adjusting to, and solving problems. Problems go on as long as living goes on and normality is adjusting to and solving the problems of living.

What mental health practitioners are all about

Mental health practitioners work with people, people who are having trouble getting along and adjusting to the stresses and demands of their situation and people who are experiencing emotional tension and distress within themselves. Mental health practitioners also work toward preventing these conditions in the first place. Thus, they are concerned with the social conditions and in helping people to learn skills for getting along and for coping with problems before they are overwhelmed by them.

In order to do these things, mental health practitioners need to know many things about people, for example, how maladjustments and emotional distress are caused. In addition, they need to develop the skills and techniques for alleviating these conditions.

From the beginning the practitioner should be aware that the skills and techniques available, while often effective, seldom produce fast, dramatic changes in people. Unlike many treatments for physical disorders in which the patient basically passively receives the treatment from someone else, in mental health the patient's desire to change and willingness to try new things are very often important if major changes are to take place. There are some pills and medicine that can be helpful in some situations, but their use is very limited unless they are combined with some of the more behavioral methods for helping the person deal with the situation.

Who are mental health practitioners?

Anyone who has ever helped a friend or a family member with some disturbing personal problem or who has soothed an upset frightened child has in a sense been a mental health practitioner. However, such activities, while common, are usually very limited in what they can deal with and, unfortunately, as often as not what is done may not be helpful. Sometimes it can be harmful.

For many years mental health practice was considered a professional field. The providers were limited to those with very specialized training and graduate degrees. But in recent years it has been found that not only are there not enough of the professional mental health workers to provide the needed service, but for many people mental health services by professionals is not what is required. A growing number of what have been called paraprofessional mental health providers are now working in a range of mental health service situations.

Professional mental health practitioners

Of the professionally trained mental health providers there is a *psychiatrist* who is a doctor of medicine and who also has had extensive training in dealing with emotionally disturbed people. In addition to other things, psychiatrists provide physical treatments for patients, such as electroshock therapy when this is indicated, and can prescribe medicines that can calm people down and help them control their feelings. The *clinical psychologist* is a doctor of philosophy who has training in the basic causes of human behavior and can, among other things, provide special therapy procedures such as behavior modification techniques, in addition to the general psychotherapeutic methods. The psychologist is usually skilled in assessing a patient's personality, intelligence, and cognitive functioning through specialized psychological test procedures. The *psychiatric social worker* has advance training in working with emotionally disturbed people and their families. They can provide, in addition to other things, specialized services to help with adjustments within the family and within the community and various other kinds of therapy support. There are also a number of other professionally trained workers who contribute special skills to the mental health field. These include *psychiatric* or *mental health nurses, vocational and rehabilitation counselors, special education specialists, occupational therapists,* and others.

New-professional (paraprofessional) mental health practitioners

As has been previously mentioned, services by professionals tend to be both in short supply and also to be less than fully effective when working with certain groups. It has been known for a number of years that poor, disadvantaged people generally have more mental health problems and more severe mental health problems than do the more advantaged groups. But the poor people tend to receive the poorest mental health services for their conditions. It is not surprising that the conditions of poverty and low social status create a great deal of stress and result in the greatest amount and the greatest severity of mental health problems for such individuals. The classical studies demonstrating the relationship between social class and mental illness are the one by Hollingshead and Redlich (1956) and the study of midtown Manhattan by Srole and others (1962).

Lower socioeconomic groups are generally underrepresented in most mental health facilities. They not only receive the poorest mental health services but also the least. Why this is so is not entirely clear. But some of the main factors seem to be that the usual services are provided by the professionals, and many poor people are reluctant to go to them in the first place. In addition, they often seem to gain little help when they do. Much of this difficulty may be due to differences in the kinds of values poor people have, as compared to how the professionals look at things, as well as to the differences in cultural backgrounds of the two groups. When poor minority people do come for services, they seem to find little benefit and seldom return. They may find it difficult to understand and trust the therapist or the method that the therapist uses. The patient may be required to reveal much personal information or the patient may be asked to look into his or her motives and reasons for doing a particular thing. Lower socioeconomic people may not understand the therapist's big words and ideas. Professional therapists simply seem strange and different. Their values and what they consider to be right or proper behavior are often totally different from that of the patient. For many poor people, this whole process may be frightening and sometimes it seems to be insulting.

Most of these difficulties, however, can be overcome when the services are provided by mental health paraprofessionals, especially when the paraprofessionals are from the same community and cultural group as the patients. The patient can feel comfortable and understood by the paraprofessionals. The paraprofessionals can understand how the patient sees things and know much more clearly what the patient's real situation in the family and the community might be. Although paraprofessionals do not have the extensive schooling of the professionals, with some background training and experience in mental health concepts and techniques they can provide effective services often in just the situations in which the more professionally oriented approach does not work well.

Paraprofessionals have been used in mental health programs in different ways and they may have a wide range of levels of training and education. In programs in which the people being served are from a culture and a socioeconomic level and even with a language which is very different from that of the dominant middle-class culture, they may be served best by paraprofessionals who come from that culture themselves, identify with it, and know the language or the street talk. Education and training levels are of less importance in such situations than are cultural relevance and understanding of and acceptance by the people. Programs dealing with individuals from Mexican-American barrios, black ghettos, or Indian reservations are examples of situations in which culturally relevant paraprofessionals would be most appropriate (Alley & Blanton, 1978).

But to be an effective paraprofessional, it is not enough to just be one of the people. It requires a certain kind of person who can be warm and understanding, who is trusted by the people, and who can relate well to others. Paraprofessionals must also have some orientation and basic training for the job.

The education and training levels of paraprofessionals range from no formal educational requirements to programs in which a university degree and very thorough skill training are required. The ability to understand and to relate to the people being served is, however, crucial to all paraprofessionals and professionals alike. Often, paraprofessionals with high-level training function well in programs serving a wide range of patients, including many from the dominant culture (Wagonfeld & Robin, 1980). At that level of training, the paraprofessionals often tend to function much in the same way as do the professionals, but they have a more limited range of methods and less responsibility. Frequently, these individuals go on for further education and train to become professionals.

What skills and abilities do mental health practitioners need?

Mental health work is basically carried out through an interpersonal relationship between the practitioner and the person needing help. Mental health practitioners thus must have or be able to develop the skills needed to develop good relationships with the people with whom they are dealing. Some of the characteristics needed are having a sincere desire to help others, being interested, liking and enjoying people and relationships, and being able to accept people without putting too much of one's own values on them. Being warm and encouraging and developing skill in understanding what it is like for the other person are important factors. Mental health relationships also involve trust. In order for the patient to share his or her private feelings and very personal behavior with someone else, the patient must feel confidence in the practitioner and trust what the practitioner will do with that information. Since confidentiality is an important aspect of the relationship, mental health practitioners must be very careful to guard the privacy of their patients within the mental health system in which they are working.

Self-knowledge is also often important. Working with the personal problems of others can be stressful because it touches the emotions and the sensitivities of the mental health worker's personality in ways that can blur the worker's ability to help the patient. The better one knows oneself, the better one can help patients.

Basic information and skills that mental health practitioners should develop

People are very complex and the factors having to do with how they came to behave the way they do and how changes can take place involve a great deal of information from very many different sources. Even so, at best our knowledge of human behavior, as of now, is still limited and there is much that is not known. In the selection of basic concepts to be covered in this book, consideration was given to topics that should provide a basic foundation for a starting level for a practitioner of mental health services. The important information areas that will be covered are described below.

Part 1. Fundamental concepts briefly

Part 1 is an orientation and a review of the important basic areas of information needed for mental health work.

The material is covered briefly since many individuals going into this work will have had some intensive courses in the subject areas and they will need only a review before getting into the clinical technique portions of the book. For those who have had little background in the field, Chapters 1 through 5 should provide a general orientation to the foundations of the clinical methods and perhaps they will suggest areas in which further study might be helpful.

Know the people and the community you serve   This chapter includes consideration of the importance of knowing the community, the people, the culture, and the values in the community in which a mental health practitioner is to work. Any methods to be used effectively must consider many factors. The relationship of people's socioeconomic levels and culture and their views of illness are important. The ways people behave, the way they think, the way they speak, and what they consider worthwhile or not worthwhile are related to the person's sociocultural experience. People from poor socioeconomic conditions may do and think about things very differently from those from a middle-class experience. Mental health practitioners with high levels of training often have difficulty understanding and working with patients who have had little education and are from poor socioeconomic conditions. Even practitioners of different levels of training and background may experience difficulties in working well together because of their differences in values and experience. Knowing how other groups think and react to things is most important.

For some groups, traditional folk healing procedures are important and should be respected. What can be learned by practitioners from folk healing will be considered.

Know yourself   Mental health practitioners have personal problems and blind spots like everyone else. The pressures and responsibilities of mental health work may also put additional strain on practitioners. It is important that the practitioners' own problems do not interfere with their being able to effectively help the people with whom they work. For these reasons, mental health practitioners must be especially aware of their own feelings and problems and must learn how to cope successfully with their own lives. This chapter considers ways in which practitioners can continue to expand their self-knowledge and their coping skills.

How people get that way—coping and adjusting to stress and frustration
Chapter 4 is a brief consideration of how human behavior develops both normally and abnormally and it describes some of the sources of stress and difficulty as well as the general means in which people try to cope with their problems. Understanding how people become the way they are is often basic to helping them to find better means of adjustments.

Recognizing the signs and types of emotional disorder   Chapter 5 considers the major types of abnormal behavior ranging from adjustments to situational stress and crisis problems through behavior disorders that are so severe that they involve the inability to deal realistically with the world. Practitioners need to know how to recognize emotional disorders in terms of their type, seriousness, and treatment indications.

Part 2. Clinical methods and techniques

Part 2 covers the basic methods of clinical intervention in some detail. The choice of methods included are considered to be both basic and those most likely to be of use in general clinical situations that beginning practitioners will find themselves dealing with.

Clinical interviewing   Interviewing is the basic tool of clinical work. It is through interviewing that most of the assessment of a patient's difficulty is done, and the interview is the basis of most treatment methods. Clinical interviewing is a fundamental skill that must be learned well because so many other clinical aspects depend on the effective use of the interview method. The techniques and the types of interviewing are discussed in Chapter 6.

Crisis treatment and suicide prevention: intervention and therapy   Chapter 7 describes a mental health treatment modality for dealing with people who are experiencing acute, intensive upsets in their lives. Working with suicidal crisis is a special aspect considered. Its goal is to help the person regain balance and control and to be able to function adequately again. It is a form of brief psychotherapy and is a procedure of choice for a large number of cases seen in active mental health clinics.

Marital and family treatment methods   Marital discord and family problems, including behavior disorders of children, are common reasons that people seek mental health help. Methods for counseling couples and family members to achieve better relationships and understanding are among the most useful and important skills for the mental health practitioner.

Problem drinking and alcoholism: Effects and treatment   Alcoholism is a widespread problem and is commonly involved in many other problems such as marital and family discord and in many crisis situations. Alcoholism is a drug addiction; it can cause grave physical damage to the body, and it can result in badly disrupted life situations for the drinker, the drinker's family, and many others as well. Treatment approaches from detoxification through various phases of counseling are covered in this chapter.

Special intervention methods briefly   Once the mental health worker has mastered some of the basic methods, he or she is perhaps ready to become acquainted with other of the many additional methods and techniques available today. Some of these are briefly covered in Chapter 10. They include the role of the patient advocate, behavioral therapy, assertiveness training, sex therapy, psychopharmacology, and a special section on knowing and dealing with the welfare and social benefits systems.

Prevention and evaluation   Preventing emotional disorders is part of the mental health worker's focus and potentially it can be the most important in the mental health program. Workers need to know what effect they are having. Therefore, evaluation procedures at all levels must be part of the total methods in doing work in this field.

1 Mental health is concerned with helping people who have difficulty adjusting in their families, socially, and at work, who are tormented within themselves, who cannot control their drinking, or who get in trouble with the law. Mental health is also concerned with the prevention of these disorders.

2 There are different ways of viewing emotional disturbance: as an illness, as internal conflict, as a sociocultural difficulty, or as a problem of living.

3 There are no clear dividing lines between what is considered normal and what is considered abnormal. Abnormality can be looked at in terms of behavior deviating from one's social or cultural group, of classical symptoms, of degrees of felt distress, or as a failure to maximize one's potential.

4 Mental health practitioners may have various levels of training, background, and professional degrees. Paraprofessionals are often particularly effective in working with certain types of disadvantaged or lower socioeconomic people because the paraprofessionals often share values and have personal familiarity with such problems.

5 Mental health workers at any level need certain basic understandings of behavior and they require specific skills and methods in order to help people. These include a knowledge of the people being served, their cultural traditions and expectations, self-knowledge, a knowledge of how behavioral patterns including maladaptive ones develop, being able to recognize maladaptive behavior forms and being able to develop skills in basic interviewing, crisis intervention, family and marital counseling, alcohol addiction counseling, and in other methods.

Know the people
and the community
you serve

A community can mean many things, but generally it refers to people who share a location in which they live and work, play, and die. Communities are made by people as well as being made up of people. Although people make the community, the community influences the lives and the behaviors of the people in the community as well. Understanding an individual's problems and dilemmas can only adequately be done by understanding where and how these matters fit into the individual's interaction with the community. A knowledge of a person's community, of its resources or what it lacks in resources, and of how the community works is essential to providing the best help for the individual in distress.

An example of how knowledge of the community is important is the case of Helen. Helen, a twelve-year-old girl, had not been attending school and was found living in a vacant house with three teen-age boys. All of them were drunk when they were found by the school's truant officer. Helen was referred to a mental health clinic by the juvenile court. In working with this situation the mental health worker's knowledge of the community, its people, and its resources was quite essential. To understand this girl, it was important first to know about her family situation, where she lived, and with whom. In this case, it turned out that she was the third of eight children living with her mother in a tiny three-room run-down house in one of the poorest sections of the community. Her mother worked long hours as a maid at a motel and was always too tired to pay attention to the children. Her father had not been heard from for years. The girl stopped going to school because it didn't interest her and because the other children teased her about her clothes and her lunch. There was always too much noise at home to study and she felt the teachers didn't like her.

The three essential things that the mental health practitioner needed to do in this case drew heavily on the worker's knowledge of the people and the community. First, the practitioner needed to know more of the home and family situation in order to determine whether help and changes there could provide this girl and her brothers and sisters with a better living situation. Second, the mental health practitioner needed to work with the courts and the juvenile probation people with regard to the best way to help. And, third, the mental health practitioner needed to contact the school and the school administrators to work on improving that situation so that school could be a satisfactory experience for the girl. Other factors, such as neighbors, church, and relatives, needed to be considered as well.

There are still additional things that a mental health practitioner should do in working with such a case. Not the least of these would be to develop a helpful, trusting relationship with the girl herself. But to do that, knowledge of her people, her values, and her community resources would be vital.

Who and what are where in the community

The physical aspects of the community include the area in which the community is contained and the locations of all the things in it. The mental health practitioner should have a good idea of the different neighborhoods within the community, the kinds of housing, and where and how different groups of people live. For instance, are there special ethnic or nationality areas? Do Greek families tend to live in one neighborhood, black families in another, or Oriental families in still another? More broadly, what are the main subgroups of the community? If there are different subgroups, it is important to know something about the background, culture, values, and customs of each of the different groups and to know how they think about things and how they are likely to behave in different situations.

The mental health practitioner should know the locations of and be in contact with the major resources of the commumity: the schools, the police, the courts, the hospitals and the doctors, the lawyers, and the probation officers. They should know where the stores and churches are, who the storekeepers and the ministers are, where the parks and playgrounds, the movie theaters, the bars, the prostitutes, and the homosexuals are, who the community leaders are, and who the community troublemakers are.

Below are listed some ways the practitioner can use to check his or her knowledge of the community to be served.

1. *Who lives where?* People often live in areas with others who are similar to themselves in ethnicity and cultural ways, religion, economic level, and maybe in style of living. Such clustering of similar people isn't always by choice. Poor people, for instance, simply have to live in the areas where housing costs the least. But others may be able to choose the neighborhood and neighbors they prefer.

A useful project is to find out where the different groups of people live in the community to be served or in one that the practitioner is interested in or knows about. The practitioner should make a rough map of the area of the community to be studied and then find out what ethnic groups live in that area. If they tend to live in a concentration with other similar people, that area should be outlined on the map. A different color pencil should be used for each group. Then, in still other colors the areas where the poorest people live and where the lowest cost housing is should be marked off. The same should be done with another color to mark off the areas of the most expensive housing. The practitioner should note whether or not young families live in different areas from the elderly.

2. *What services are available and where are they?* The practitioner should list the available services that people can use. Learning what is available and what isn't is the first step. The services should include such things as churches, hospitals and clinics, nursing homes, children's day-care centers, police and sheriff, legal services, transportation, schools and universities, stores and businesses, entertainment areas such as movies, recreational centers, sports facilities, parks, bars, and so on. These and many more should be known and indicated on the map. Of course, they will be different from community to community. The locations of these services should be shown on the map by means of symbols. A different symbol should be used for each type of service. For example, a cross may be used to indicate a Christian church. One thing that may become clear in doing this is which groups of people live most conveniently to what kinds of services. The map will also indicate which services may be difficult

for some groups to get to. It also may show which services are needed in what areas.

3. *Where are the trouble spots in the community?* It often turns out that certain areas of the community have higher crime rates than others. The local police can usually locate such places and can indicate what kinds of crime occur where. Areas where drunkenness and disturbances are more likely to occur, where there are frequent family fights, where delinquent children most often are found, or where most physical sickness is found should be shown on the map.

4. *Who are the community leaders?* Community leaders are not just the official government leaders. Often some of the more influential leaders of a community are the people in the neighborhoods whom others respect and listen to. These are the people members of the community often go to with their problems and for advice. They may be neighbors, ministers or priests, folk healers, or labor union officers. Knowing who these individuals are and developing contacts with them can prove useful in helping with many kinds of problem situations of patients.

The different areas marked on the map should soon show a pattern and tell some important things about the community. For instance, is the high crime rate located in the poorest housing sections where also much of the drunkenness takes place? Are the best schools and shopping conveniences located near the best housing? Looking for such patterns on a map may be very helpful in learning about the community and how it operates, and even more so, it may suggest some possible solutions to community problems.

The examples given above are only a few ways in which this mapping location procedure may help in learning about the community to be served. There are, of course, many other services than the ones mentioned and perhaps particular key things that are necessary but are lacking in a given community. The mapping procedure must be tailored for each individual community. The ways to find out what groups and services exist and how to locate them are many. The sources can be people who have lived a long time in the community, government records, the census report, policemen and mailmen, teachers, and many others. In doing such a mapping project of the community, it is important that the practitioner use as many sources as possible and be original in finding the needed information.

Every community is different and unique. It may have things that were not mentioned above or they may be in different combinations. The mental health provider should know and understand the community, for in this way he or she can best serve the people.

Knowing the people in the community

Some communities are made up of a number of different subgroups, each of which does some things differently and values things in very different ways. Other communities are made up of people who basically share the same background, values, and traditions. It is essential in working in a community to know and understand the culture, the traditions, the beliefs, and the values of each element of the community.

Social class: Ethnicity and behavioral styles

Poverty and behavioral characteristics

People's behaviors and personalities are affected both by the culture and the ethnic group from which they come and by the social class level that characterizes their social and economic status. These factors can be very influential and should be considered in every case. Cultural, ethnic, and social class level factors show themselves in terms of the beliefs that people hold, their values about most of the important things in their lives, and even in the ways they reason and think. Furthermore, these factors are reflected in the way people use language, how they react to situations, how they express their feelings and emotions, how they are likely to deal with problems, and even to whom they turn for help. While each culture and ethnic group provides some things which contribute to special ways of behaving, and to particular values and beliefs, the social class level (social and economic status) is also related to a person's values and behavioral styles.

Some people even argue that social class factors may be more important than ethnic and cultural factors. It has been observed, for instance, that poor people generally have many behavioral similarities regardless of what ethnic group or culture they come from. Oscar Lewis (1966) has called poverty a culture itself and refers to it as the culture of poverty.

Lewis has studied the personality characteristics of the poor, especially individuals from some very economically impoverished Mexican villages. Some of the most important aspects of personality and behavior which Lewis says are characteristic of the poor are as follows:

1. The poor have a strong present-time orientation. That is, they tend, more so than other groups of people, to live in the here-and-now. They are not particularly concerned with what has happened in the past and in some ways are not influenced by their previous experiences in the sense that they may seem not to learn from their mistakes or to capitalize on or take advantage of their successes. In this same sense, there is relatively little attention given to the future or sometimes no great concern for what the long-range consequences of their immediate behavior might bring. Thus, the idea of sacrificing and saving now for a better tomorrow is not a very strong value for them. Rather, the orientation is more likely to be enjoy what you have now while you can.

This present-time orientation is not at all surprising. People who must exist on very little have nothing to save to begin with, and they have little to look forward to in the future. Their experience has not shown them that it would be beneficial to sacrifice for the future. Instead, their experience suggests that if you happen to have something you had better enjoy it now because it may well be that it will not be there at all tomorrow.

2. Along with the present-time orientation, according to Lewis, there also appears to be comparatively little ability or desire to defer and to delay gratification. The circumstances of the poor seldom provide great benefits for delaying gratification or holding off until later. Generally speaking, then, with the poor there is more premarital sex, more of what appears to middle-class people to be self-indulgent kinds of behaviors, and perhaps more direct pleasure-seeking than in groups in better financial circumstances.

Both the tendency to live in the here-and-now and the lesser likelihood of delaying gratification are related to another tendency, that of little planning ahead and looking to the future. But the poor, after all, do not have much of a future to plan toward.

3. A sense of resignation and fatalism is also a characteristic described by Lewis. There is a general feeling among poor people that they have little or no control over what happens to them

and that nothing can be done about their difficult circumstances and fate. They may feel that that's the way it is or is supposed to be. This attitude may partly explain why the poor often seem to accept such intolerable conditions and why they do not seek and demand change and improvement.

4. The poor have a higher tolerance for psychological pathology of all sorts than do others. They accept and are willing to live with a great deal more disturbed behavior of others within the family and community than other social groups might. For instance, such things as alcoholism among family members, beating wives and girlfriends, antisocial behavior, and criminal acts are usually more tolerated among the poor than they are among other groups.

5. The poor also tend to be generally outgoing, to be friendly, warm, open people who enjoy others. They are close to their nuclear families and they tend to have many open, friendly, social interactions with their own people. To outsiders, however, sometimes they may seem very closed and hostile.

6. The poor also tend to be much more oriented toward authority, power, and control than are the nonpoor. Authority is feared, often resented, but where it is strong it is obeyed. The father, when present, usually plays a very dominant authoritarian role in the family. There is often much fear-based respect for the powers in the neighborhood, such as juvenile gangs, the police, and the welfare system.

7. Some other factors included in the notion of the culture of poverty are impulsiveness, that is, acting immediately and directly without much thought or concern for the consequences, and a tendency to think in fairly concrete, realistic terms rather than in more abstract ways.

8. The language of the poor has been described as restricted, relatively undifferentiated, and simple. It is said to be lacking in modifiers, to be not too precise, and to be aimed at supporting the social structure rather than providing information.

9. Another factor is a general feeling of inferiority and low self-esteem, which seems to be quite common among the poor.

It should be kept in mind that these characteristics are not necessarily true of every person from an economically impoverished background.

In fact, further research studies have not generally given a great deal of support to Lewis' factors being characteristic of the poor. However, the research has been done in such a way that it is not possible to really say whether or not these characteristics truly describe the poor.

Studies have shown, however, that lower social class individuals, in comparison with higher, do show less of a motivation toward achieving and that they tend generally to have less of a sense that they are in control of their fate. Rather, they tend to feel more controlled from the outside. Poverty seems to produce a sense of defeat and apathy which in turn leads to an attitude of "what is the use of trying." As compared to middle-class people, poor people tend to respond better to rewards which are tangible and from others, and they are less likely to do something because they think it is the right and proper thing to do.

When providing mental health services for people from the culture of poverty it is useful to bear these characteristics in mind. But since the characteristics obviously do not fit everyone, they must be considered carefully and cautiously. It is suggested that the mental health practitioner might do best to work with people with these characteristics in the here-and-now and without being overly concerned about lessons from past behavior. Goals that are far in the future are not too likely to be important motivators. Guidance might have to be fairly specific, perhaps rather directive and authoritarian, but done in an atmosphere of social warmth, acceptance, and friendliness. It should be communicated in simple direct words.

Middle-class behavioral characteristics and personality styles

Just as poverty seems to influence people's values and personality styles, so does membership in the higher social and economic brackets. In some important ways, middle-class values and styles of thinking and doing things can be very different from those of the poor. It is not surprising, then, that people from middle- and lower-socioeconomic backgrounds may have difficulty understanding each other. Often they have different expectations, value different things, or may even become enthused or upset by opposite occurrences. Certainly, when mental health workers with middle-class values deal with individuals with the value system of the culture of poverty, knowledge and respect for the poor people's ways of thinking and doing things are essential if a good helping relationship is to be established.

It is equally necessary that mental health providers from backgrounds that are not middle-class are aware of middle-class value systems and behavioral styles. Since almost all professionals come from middle-class backgrounds or have, through their schooling and positions, taken on middle-class values, the other mental health service providers in the system need to be aware of how the professionals think and how they prefer to do things. This is important because the professionals usually have great influence and power in mental health delivery systems. In addition, most government agencies that fund mental health service programs for the poor are very middle class in their orientation and expectations.

Some of the most impoortant middle-class characteristics are listed below:

1. The middle-class time perspective, in contrast to the present-time orientation of the culture of poverty, is generally geared toward the future. The middle-class, which includes the professionals, are generally future oriented. They are concerned about what will happen next and they plan for future developments and events.

2. The importance and value that middle-class people place on the future are related to a characteristic behavior of delaying present gratifications and pleasures so that they might have more and better later on. Professionals, for example, have been willing and able to delay immediate pleasures in order to complete long periods of schooling and training. They do this in order to prepare for a future income and occupation. This often has meant considerable restrictions on dating, delayed marriage, early restricted income, and much effort expended on hard work and study.

3. Middle-class people generally have a considerably greater sense of being able to control and to determine their own futures than do the poor. Professionals especially have been trained to have a strong sense of responsibility about using approved methods, keeping accurate and detailed records, and following up on cases. They expect that everyone else should also do things this way and they are often amazed and frustrated because these things are not as important to others as they are to them.

4. Middle-class people often tend to be more socially reserved or inhibited in their relationships than are the poor. They may be less friendly, less outgoing, and less able to relate openly. It usually takes longer to get to know them and they may never relate with the same friendly closeness that the poor do.

5. Among their own middle-class groups they generally tend to treat each other on an equal accepting basis. However, some

may regard those from the culture of poverty, those with less education and money, as being much less knowledgeable and find that they behave in ways they do not consider entirely proper and acceptable. They may take a condescending, almost parental kind of authoritarian stance with regard to such individuals.

6. Middle-class people generally do not tolerate deviant behavior, be it abnormal psychological reactions, alcohol and drug abuse, family violence, or delinquent or criminal behavior. They generally tend to be moralistic about such things.

7. Middle-class people, especially the professionals, often think in more abstract terms than in concrete, specific, everyday terms. Their language and their ideas may involve complicated words and ideas which are not always in touch with feelings and everyday occurrences. Generally, middle-class people see themselves as representing the proper standards of values and behavior and they have an air of smug confidence.

8. Middle-class people are very achievement oriented and ambitious and they are highly motivated to get ahead and to gain success, especially in terms of money, power, and admiration by others. They are more guided by their internal values and beliefs than they are by what happens in the world around them.

But as with the culture of poverty, there are large differences among middle-class individuals. One should always be alert to the fact that what is said here about the middle-class does not apply to every individual who happens to be middle-class or a professional.

Dealing with different value systems: Professionals and paraprofessionals

Most people grow up learning certain values, beliefs, and styles of behaviors. Generally they are comfortable with them, and it may not even occur to them that anything else could or should be done or viewed differently. Since most people stay within their own social groups, they may face little interaction with those of different values.

However, children from the culture of poverty who are taught by middle-class teachers obviously experience this clash of values. Their teachers are also confronted with these value differences. Mental health professionals trying to work with patients from a culture of poverty also face a wide variation in values and styles of behaviors. This may be an important factor in explaining why many professionals are relatively unsuccessful in helping poor people.

Similarly, paraprofessionals who come from the culture of poverty and who must interact with middle-class professionals face the same difficulties. Since very often it is the middle-class professionals who have the power in the system, the paraprofessionals have a large stake in trying to understand the orientation and the values of the professionals.

Both professionals and paraprofessionals should openly recognize the differences in their values. They should discover which things are important in each other's social class value system and what things each considers most important for helping the patient. Good communication, wanting to do the best possible job, and cooperation are essential.

By and large, the system in which paraprofessionals work is a system developed by and paid for by the middle-class, even though it is often aimed toward help for people of poverty level. It is crucial that paraprofessionals understand the values and the demands of the general social system and how it operates. Professionals often see themselves as representing that system, and they feel that because of their training and professional position they are the ones who should have the authority and final decision power. When this is the case, the paraprofessionals may well feel depreciated, powerless, and resentful.

It is our position that the best relationship between paraprofessional and professional is one of open communication and acknowledgment of the differences in values. Each is there because of a special contribution he or she has to offer the patient. On one hand, the paraprofessional is on the firing line; the paraprofessional has the skills for relating to and to understanding the patient in ways the professional usually cannot. On the other hand, the professional has special technical knowledge in methods (for example, specialized means of therapy, medications, psychological tests, and the knowledge of procedures in the system, such as how to hospitalize an individual) which the paraprofessional will need. The professional can provide consultation and advice, but the paraprofessional must be open to them and be willing to receive them. Most importantly, the paraprofessional must recognize when he or she is in need of professional input and special methods. Experience and being open, not defensive, are keys to a productive relationship.

The professional, for his or her part, must recognize the paraprofessional's special skills, special knowledge, and capacity to reach patients. The paraprofessional has the most difficult job with the most difficult cases and has not had the luxury of the long training of the professional.

Respect for the skill and for the sensitivity of the paraprofessionals and an understanding of their value differences are perhaps the keys to successful professional consultation with paraprofessionals. If the professional conveys respect and a willingness to understand and attempts to apply his or her knowledge and skills in ways that the paraprofessional can use, then the professional's contribution can be great. Professionals who feel that their role is basically one of supervision, control, and direction may well depreciate the role of the paraprofessional, and such an attitude can interfere with effective case management. In some cases, the paraprofessional may have to help the professional recognize and deal with this problem.

Cultural beliefs about illness and cure

Beliefs about the causes of emotional problems and beliefs about how these problems can be treated and cured are of particular importance to mental health workers. Many people do not fully share the current scientific views on the cause of illness; instead, they hold to more traditional ideas from older cultures. Part of understanding these people is understanding their beliefs and indeed respecting them, and sometimes even using them in treatment.

Concept of illness and respect for folk healing

Only recently has it been recognized that a very important factor in a person's response to psychological treatment methods is what that person believes is the cause of illness because that is what indicates by whom and by what means the person believes he or she can be helped. People educated in Western industrialized cultures generally have a scientific view of the causes and treatments for mental illness. Even within this scientific realm, however, there are divergent scientific explanations and treatment methods for mental disorders. These range from the constitutional and physical theories and the biochemical theories to a wide variety of psychological theories such as the dynamic or the learning theory approaches. There is reason to believe that a person responds to a given therapy approach when the approach represents attitudes and explanations about the causes and cure of the behavior that the patient finds consistent with his or her own beliefs and can accept. Perhaps a crucial element of therapy is convincing an individual that the method being used is the one that that person requires.

Common factors in scientific and folk healing

Frank (1973) has pointed out basic commonalities among successful healers which transcend method. These common factors apply not only to the scientifically based approaches but also to religious and folk healing. These factors start with the severe anxiety and despair that the patient is experiencing. To be effective, the healer must provide confidence and instill hope in the individual. In order to be able to do that, the healer must, in the patient's eyes, possess qualities which include the power to produce change, a similar outlook on illness as the patient, and a manner of doing things that is acceptable to the patient. It is important that the healer and patient are similar in background, values, and aspirations. The healer's ability to influence the patient comes from the healer's having the same attitudes and values as the patient's family and cultural group, basically all that is important to the patient. When the patient feels this kind of acceptance and understanding of his or her basic values and views, the patient can believe in the power of the healer and can develop an expectation of help and relief from such an individual. The healer's personal attributes can then be used effectively with methods that are in terms of culture and values acceptable to the patient. The method that the healer uses from then on must be consistent with the values and assumptions about illness and treatment that both patient and healer share. In addition, the method and goals must be consistent with the cultural expectations of the setting in which the patient belongs or wishes to belong.

Who shares traditional beliefs?

In many settings in which patients come from cultural and ethnic groups which in recent times have practiced or follow the traditions of religious or folk healing it is very possible that many patients will share such traditional beliefs about the causes and cure of disorders. This is even more likely if the patient has had relatively little education in Western schools or if the individual closely identifies with his or her traditional culture. These beliefs may be pervasive and enduring, and they may exist along with scientific views. For example, the author knows a trained nurse of American Indian descent who believes that the medicine men of her tribe often can cure people whom Western doctors have been unable to cure. Furthermore, she herself goes to a medicine man for help but she also follows the instructions of western doctors when she is ill.

It is the author's impression that in the generally traditional Indian tribe with which he has worked that almost all tribal members share the belief of their tribe's cultural concept of illness and its shamanistic approach to cure. There are, of course, degrees of commitment to these beliefs. Many who have had more formal education and experience elsewhere probably hold the belief less intensely than those who have not. The point is that in working in mental health with such a group, treatment techniques based on Western scientific concepts may be very limited in application. Often the more effective approach is one that acknowledges and also works within the cultural belief system of the individual concerned.

It is our impression that belief in and acceptance of these cultural and religious views of illness and cure are much more pervasive than is generally recognized by those trained in Western mental health techniques. American blacks, for instance, have a definite heritage in tribal Africa and perhaps have been influenced as well by West Indian voodoo. Among Mexican-Americans a bad witch who causes disorders among the people is countered by a *curandero*, a person who is capable of diagnosing the evil spells and providing means for overcoming them. Since early times the Christian faith has considered faith healing a part of the religion. Faith healing is increasingly being practiced today.

Treatment programs based on these cultural and religious belief systems can and indeed do have powerful effects on people who basically share the assumptions of that system and have faith in both the system and the healer representing the system. The effectiveness of such approaches has been shown with both physical and with more purely psychological disorders.

As Frank has pointed out, the effectiveness of such procedures probably rests on most of the same basic principles as the effectiveness of more Western scientifically based healing procedures for psychological problems. A key element for both is that the method of cure must be consistent with the belief system of the person with the disorder. When the healer's assumptions and methods are in conflict with the patient's belief system, or when the patient has serious doubts about what is being done, the possibilities of treatment progress are probably poor. The healer's power and ability to convince the patient that his or her method will work sometimes can themselves bring about a change. But we suspect that often when there is poor progress in treatment, especially when the patient does not do what the treatment system requires or does not return for appointments (as is frequently the case with lower socioeconomic patients), it is because the patient does not share the therapist's beliefs about the cause and cure of the disorder. The patient has not been convinced of the power of the method used to help him or her.

Beliefs about how illness is caused

In traditional and tribal societies physical or psychological illnesses are usually not considered separately. The causes of any illness or even any life disruptions are basically tied to the group's religious beliefs. Thus, the illness may be seen as coming directly from the gods or the spirits as a punishment for breaking tribal taboos or as a result of having offended the spirits of animals or other things that are considered sacred by the group. In other cases, the cause of the illness may be seen as stemming from the evil magic performed by individuals with certain powers who have chosen the sick person as their victim.

Types of magic   Some of the common means by which spells are thought to be put upon victims are by *contagious magic, imitative magic,* and *projective magic.* Contagious magic refers to casting a spell on an individual's footprint or clothing or obtaining something that was once part of the victim's body, such as hair, fingernail clippings, or even feces and urine. With possession of such intimate material from the person, the one having the evil power can cast a spell on the victim and create the difficulty. In some cultures in which this belief is held, people are extremely concerned and careful about secretly burying their feces, old clothes, and anything that could be used for this purpose.

Imitative magic refers to the method whereby an image or a little doll, perhaps of straw or some other material, is made of the person. The illness is thought to be caused when the image or doll is hurt in some way. Pins put in various places or burning or choking the image or doll result in the victim's experiencing sharp stabbing pains, burning sensations, or choking sensations.

Projective magic refers to the one having the evil power pointing an object such as a sharpened bone or a spear toward the body of the victim. The victim may be many miles away, but as a result of this pointing and other ritual and magical acts, the victim experiences a penetration of his or her body by the unseen pointed object. Victims have been known to die when they have been convinced that this has happened.

There are a number of other beliefs about methods used to inflict illness on victims. In most cultures there is a prescribed way in which this happens and often a prescribed reason for it happening. Violating a taboo or rule of the group is an example. Usually, each society also has its people who are designated as healers and established methods to provide the cure. The accepted healer can determine what has caused the illness in terms of the culture's concept of the illness and has the powers and rituals to provide the cure.

Some of the traditional beliefs of two tribal cultures are briefly reviewed below. Whenever these beliefs are strongly held, the traditional healer, either the medicine man or shaman, is obviously the proper one to treat those believing in them.

For many individuals from such backgrounds these beliefs, although not primary, still are held along with the more western and scientific beliefs. Sometimes the treatment must deal with the problem at both levels.

While it is not very likely that the mental health practitioner will ever come across patients with these beliefs in pure form, knowing how they can operate extends understanding of those patients who in part hold some level of such beliefs. Some of the traditional healing patterns of an American Indian tribe and of Australian Aborigines are briefly discussed below.

An American Indian tribe's concept of illness and cure   The traditional Papago beliefs and practices with regard to illness are generally similar to those of other tribal groups (Kahn, Williams, Galvez, Lejero, Conrad, & Goldstein, 1975). It is of interest that although the Papagos are largely Catholic and have been for over a hundred years, their religion in fact is probably a blend of continuing traditional beliefs and Catholicism. The traditional Papago belief is that illness is caused either by evildoers who cast spells on people or by the ailing person who has sometimes even unknowingly offended spirits in the natural surroundings. The medicine man has the power to diagnose the offending cause. It is of note that among the Papagos there is some specialization. One kind of medicine man specializes in determining the cause of the disorder and another kind of medicine man specializes in the cure. The diagnostic medicine man can determine the nature of the illness through such methods as how smoke blown over the patient curls and by waving sacred eagle feathers. The cure, or Papago sing, is a ritual in which the healing medicine man goes through various rituals and chants sacred healing songs. He will also prescribe herbs and potions, dietary changes, and special rites the patient must carry out.

The specific form of illness or disorder is related to the specific natural spirit that was offended. Offending the tarantula spirit can cause pain in the ear; offending the turtle can cause difficulty in walking. Similarly, offending the horned toad causes pain in the joints and offending the deer causes severe headaches. The owl is feared as the spirit of a person returning from the dead. It is interesting that persons who have committed suicide are said to belong to the devil and that their spirits return as devil spirits trying to capture their relatives for the devil's purposes.

An Australian Aborigine's concept of illness and healing   According to
Elkin (1974), the traditional Australian aboriginal belief is that illness,
death, and even accidents are caused by magical or mystical actions. It
is a belief very similar to that of the Papago. Such bad happenings are
also believed to be the work of either evil sorcerers or spirits who use
magical means to cause the illness or death. One method the sorcerer
uses is to steal kidney fat from the victim or other special tissues from
internal organs in secret operations that are unknown to the victim.
The sorcerers almost always are found to be from another tribe and the
victim's tribe itself must arrange for revenge against this bad person.

But the most powerful and most feared way of causing distress for
the aborigine is that of projective magic. In this magic an evil one points
a bone or similar object toward the body of the victim and performs the
proper singing ritual. The victim experiences a penetration of his or her
body no matter how far away the victim is. Persons who feel they are
the target of such an action have been known to die as a result, the so-
called voodoo death.

When an individual suffers from an infliction or when death occurs,
the medicine man is called to decide the type of magic that was used
and to withdraw it from the sick person. The medicine man determines
who worked the bad magic and then the tribe seeks some satisfaction
by means prescribed by the culture. This may be a revenge raid on the
offender's tribe.

It should be noted that there is much danger to the person who puts
such magic into operation. For if he is not fully qualified and makes the
slightest error in the ritual, he may cause damage to the wrong person
or even to himself. Thus, this power is not used loosely.

The aborigine medicine man performs both diagnostic and curing
functions. He also holds inquests to find the source of the sorcery. In
this culture, too, specific illnesses are caused by specific forms of magic.
Rheumatism is the result of bone pointing, internal pains the result of
projection of pieces of quartz, and death the result of the patient's soul
having been stolen or spirited away. The medicine man uses a specific
ritual and formula in the area of the pain and produces the offending
bone or quartz or catches or returns the dying man's soul.

In both cultures, the Papago and the Australian aborigine, these
beliefs are deeply engrained and practiced by many of the people.
Others do not believe in them so strongly. Nevertheless, everyone
seems to believe in them to some degree and the medicine men and
their practices are deeply respected, feared, and held in awe by the
people. In both of these mental health programs respect and understanding of these traditional beliefs were basic to working within the
culture and reaching the people. In the Papago program there was an
active cooperation with the medicine men and frequent referrals to

them and from them were made. The Australian aboriginal group was detribalized and in an urban area. Thus this cooperation was less possible, but it is certainly an approach to be developed when feasible.

Aboriginal and Western beliefs

Although these Papago and Australian aboriginal belief systems about the cause and cure of illnesses may seem strange or even ridiculous to those brought up to believe in Western scientific methods and explanations, these belief systems often do work for those who share these cultures and beliefs. Indeed, within the recent history of Western science many different methods have been proposed to treat mental illness. Often these methods seemed to work in the beginning while the proponents of them were enthusiastic and believed they worked. The use of electric shock treatment for all manner of mental disorders is an example. Now shock treatment seems effective only for severe depression. Currently, a number of so-called scientific treatment methods that are based on very different assumptions on what causes the disorders and that use very different means of treatment report similar positive rates of cure. How can these opposite and different treatment methods all be right and work? Is the factor of belief in an approach or method that is consistent with, that affirms one's belief about current illness, and that is consistent with one's cultural beliefs a necessary condition for effective treatment? From this standpoint, the traditional treatment methods of tribal groups indeed may not be so much different in these respects from the Western scientific approach. Similarly, the beliefs, rituals, and ceremonies of Western religions have many parallels to those of the tribal aboriginal peoples.

Mental health practitioners should be alert to the cultural traditions and beliefs about the causes and treatment of illness of the people with whom they work. It may be that, in some cases at least, the patient will be better served by working in some cooperative arrangement with folk healers and other practitioners of these beliefs than with Western methods. Arranging for consultation with folk healing practitioners and developing a relationship with them to augment referrals and communication can sometimes prove very useful. Of course, sound judgment is required in making such arrangements and decisions.

summary

1 Knowledge of the community in which the client lives is essential to providing the best treatment.

2 Mental health practitioners need to know in detail the characteristics of the community they serve: who lives where, what services are available and where they are, where the trouble spots are, and who the leaders are.

3 It is useful to map the information about the community in terms of locations of people, services, and activities.

4 One view suggests that personality and behavior are affected by economic and social class factors. Poverty itself has been called a culture that supposedly has distinctive personality attributes associated with it.

5 The chronically poor are said to be present-time oriented, unable to defer gratification, fatalistic, and more likely to accept psychopathology than are middle-class people.

6 Middle-class people, who include many of the mental health professionals, are future oriented, more likely to delay gratification for future gain, better able to control their fate, and to be much less tolerant of psychopathology.

7 Since professional mental health personnel are much more likely to be in charge of mental health services, it is as important for the less extensively trained personnel to understand middle-class characteristics as it is for the professionals to understand the characteristics of lower socioeconomic background patients and staff.

8 Mental health workers must be knowledgeable about various cultural values and beliefs about illness and cure. Many patients come from cultures in which folk cures are accepted. It appears that treatment methods must be consistent with the patient's belief about the cause and cure in order to be most effective. Traditional helping methods may be effective in certain cases.

9   Beliefs about causes and methods of cure of two tribal cultures, Papago Indians and Australian aborigines, were described. It was suggested that their treatment methods and certain Western scientific treatment methods are based on similar principles.

Know yourself

3

Importance for mental health workers to know themselves

Mental health work deals with people's misery and suffering, with their poor living conditions, family tragedies and difficulties, and personal defeats. This means that sometimes the most intense and rawest of feelings are involved.

Since clients come to the mental health worker with their difficulties and entrust the worker with the most private and intimate details of their lives, in many cases, the mental health worker receives the heavy burden of their clients' anguish and desperation, hopes, and fears. This can be, and not infrequently, is a source of emotional stress for the mental health worker. It is stressful because it is a very normal human response to hurt and suffer with the suffering of others. The process of helping often involves empathetically sharing, at least at a low level, the hurt and pain of the individual the mental health practitioner is trying to help. If the practitioner allows himself or herself to be too deeply drawn into the patient's experience (and sometimes it is very difficult to avoid doing so), the mental health practitioner may experience both the suffering and the strain. If this happens, the worker's effectiveness can be seriously reduced, both because of the decreased efficiency resulting from the worker's own emotional upset, and more importantly, because the mental health worker no longer can see problems from enough distance to put them in the proper perspective needed to work toward the best solutions.

Such a situation is most likely to occur when the kinds of problems or characteristics of the patient are such that they overstimulate a vulnerable emotional area for the mental health worker. If the patient and his or her problem inflame a sensitive area of the mental health practitioner's personality or life situation, the potential for emotional stress and strain on the mental health practitioner increases and the practitioner's ability to help the patient effectively decreases. Because of the intense intimate and personal relationship that the mental health worker may often have with a client, the mental health worker must be aware of and must be prepared to deal with the situation.

Pitfalls of counseling those with whom the mental health worker has personal or social relationships

While it is important for mental health workers to be sensitive, aware, and even able to experience at some level what the patients experience in order to fully understand what it is like for their patients, it is also necessary that the workers at the same time maintain an objective, realistic view of the situation to best help their patients find realistic solutions to their difficulties. For this reason, it is difficult for a mental health worker to be an effective therapist with close family members or with those with whom they have close social or personal relationships. The worker's own personal emotional involvements and needs may be so strong that they blind the worker to what is realistically going on. Furthermore, when the worker is too personally involved, it is difficult for him or her to see that his or her involvement sometimes is part of the problem. Below is an example of this situation:

Samuel, a paraprofessional mental health worker, has lived with his girlfriend, Marge, for about a year. In the past six months there have been increasing tension and disagreement between Samuel and Marge. Samuel has also been uncomfortable at work and his performance and effectiveness have been much less than they were. Samuel began drinking more heavily than usual and also began meeting various girls in bars. Marge felt hurt, rejected, neglected, and angry. The arguments increased in number and intensity. Samuel's view of the situation was that Marge was so difficult and hard to get along with that she was the main cause of his drinking and turning to other women. He felt that she complained and nagged and that he did what he did in order to get away from her demandingness. In fact, Samuel concluded that it was Marge who had personality problems and that she required counseling, which he tried to provide. His approach was to try to get her to accept the relationship problem as her own fault, suggesting that as soon as she stopped being so upset and complaining about Samuel's behavior all would be well again. Marge tried to hide her feelings for awhile, but as might be expected, this did not work out. She finally sought help from an outside counselor who did not know either of them before they sought his help.

The point of this case is that Samuel and Marge were so involved with each other emotionally that the distance and objectivity needed in order to help with their problem just couldn't be achieved when Samuel tried to counsel Marge. It required a counselor who was much less personally involved.

As this case turned out, Samuel, with the help of counseling, was able to understand what he was really doing. He was using Marge as an excuse to justify his drinking and chasing other women. He also began to recognize that his feelings for Marge were no longer as strong as they had been. Marge learned to trust her own views and values about herself much more. She felt that she would not accept Samuel's view that she was the one always at fault in their difficulties and she would not put up with Samuel's behavior. Marge was able to confront Samuel with this and left him when he refused to stop seeing other girls.

To be most effective, mental health practitioners need to have themselves reasonably well together. That is not to say that they need to be more human. Problems and adjusting to them are always present and are an ongoing aspect of everyone's life. But people in the mental health field must be in touch with their own feelings and be aware of their own sensitivities and areas of vulnerability, probably more so than do people in other fields of work. For the better mental health workers know themselves, the better they can avoid the pitfalls of overidentifying with their patients and their problems or, sometimes just as bad, being defensively unresponsive to them.

Other common pitfalls of personal involvement

Some of the most common pitfalls in this area of mental health work include overidentifying with the patient's problem. In this case, a mental health worker may come to feel almost as if the patient's problems were his or her own, to hurt for them, and to try to manage the patient's life in terms of how the mental health worker reacts to such hurt instead of helping the patient to find reasonable solutions to the situation and to work out his or her best solution. In this same vein, a mental health worker may sometimes develop very close personal intimate feelings toward the person he or she is helping on the basis of his or her own needs. If these are feelings of love and sexual attraction, the mental health worker's ability to help the patient may well be lost in the concern and striving for a more personally gratifying social or love relationship. If the feelings of the mental health practitioner are a personal dislike or anger, then the helping relationship can be defeated by a negative relationship and result in less than helpful guidance from the therapist.

None of this is completely avoidable because mental health practitioners are first human beings. Self-knowledge and knowing what he or she is sensitive to and to what kinds of things he or she reacts can be important in aiding the mental health practitioner avoid or lessen the effect of some of the situations mentioned above. Not only that, self-knowledge is important to any individual in a broader way, for it can help the individual avoid pitfalls in other relationships and situations.

Thus, self-knowledge and using that knowledge for more effective functioning, whether in mental health work as such or in life in general, is one aspect of maturity and a well-functioning individual. People can never be free of personal reactions and biases, but they can be alerted to them and reduce their effects. The better mental health practitioners know themselves and are willing to look at themselves and their behavior, the better they can decide what is realistic and in the interest of their patients and what is not.

How can one get more in touch with oneself?

Getting better acquainted with oneself can serve many purposes. Just being alert to the fact that one is sensitive to a particular thing or upset about a particular aspect of life can be useful. The primary source of self-knowledge is the individual himself or herself.

The know yourself inventory

The Know Yourself Inventory on pages 42–43 is a general guide to help people take a look into how they feel about a number of aspects of themselves and their lives. The Know Yourself Inventory asks people to think about a number of aspects about themselves and to say how they feel about those things. It will probably be most useful for an individual to complete the Know Yourself Inventory before considering the implications of the results. It can very usefully be used by an individual for his or her own guidance and kept private from others. Sharing it with a therapist and discussing the meanings of some of the individual's views with an outside person trained in these matters may in some cases be of much further use.

How to analyze the know yourself inventory

After you have completely answered all the questions in the Inventory, analyze the Inventory as follows:

1. Look over your answers. What do they tell you about yourself? If you have not been too defensive about what you have said, your answers should tell you a lot about what you think and how you feel about yourself as an individual.

2. Consider your opinions about yourself. How do they really compare with the facts? Are you, for instance, as good looking, or as poor looking, or as average as you seem to think? Consider each question in that manner.

3. On which of the items does your opinion of yourself seem realistic? How can you check whether or not the way you see yourself is the way that other people see you?

4. On which things are your feelings about yourself not supported by the facts? What is involved in your inaccurate views of yourself?

5. Consider what things you can do to change those things that you don't like about yourself now. Consider your strongest points and how they can work to make you more effective.

6. After considering all your answers, it is up to you to take action if you feel it is needed and you want to do it. Some individuals may wish to seek help from others. Knowing what the problems are is the first step to solving them.

Some ways of checking out how accurate your feelings about yourself are include finding out how others see you in this respect. Sometimes just paying closer attention to how people actually are responding to you in your everyday situations can be informative. Sometimes talking such things over with someone you feel close to or with someone you can confide in may help, although often it is best to have such discussions in a professional setting with professionals who can be more neutral and objective about these things. Some individuals go into psychotherapy to enhance their self-understanding. Many of the self-actualizing and encounter group techniques are effective in this regard.

Know Yourself Inventory

I. Who am I? (Write down your first thoughts and impressions about who you are.)

II. How do I feel about myself with regard to? (Write down your feelings about each of the following aspects of yourself.)

    a. Intelligence

    b. Appearance

    c. Physical body

    d. Attractiveness to the opposite sex

    e. Ability as a lover

    f. Ability to make friends

    g. Ability to get along with people

    h. Ability to get along with my boss

    i. The kind of husband or wife I am

    j. The kind of boyfriend or girlfriend I am

    k. The kind of mother or father I am

    l. The kind of child I am to my parents

    m. The kind of sister or brother I am

    n. The kind of friend I am

    o. The kind of enemy I am

III. List all your good points.

IV. List all your bad points.

V. What kind of people do you like or best get along with?

VI. What kind of people do you dislike or not get along with?

VII. What do you want out of life?

VIII. Why are you doing the kind of work (or other things) you do?

IX. How do you feel about the following?

    a. Alcoholics

    b. Drug addicts

    c. Disobedient children

    d. Sexual deviants

    e. Juvenile delinquents

    f. Crazy people

    g. Mental defectives

summary

1 Because mental health workers deal with feelings, anguish, hurt, and desperation they often face more than usual personal emotional stress and can get caught up in their patients' conflicts.

2 It is very difficult to remain realistic about their clients' problems when the practitioners themselves become too emotionally involved. For this reason, it is particularly difficult for a practitioner to work effectively with someone with whom he or she has a close personal relationship.

3 Self-knowledge about their own feelings and ways of reacting can assist mental health workers to be more effective with their clients and in their own lives. The Know Yourself Inventory is the way to start a personal appraisal and to increase self-understanding.

How people get that way: Coping and adjusting to stress and frustration

Development and causes of behavior

Human life starts when the sperm of the father, which carries half of the heredity of the child, penetrates the egg of the mother, which carries the other half of the hereditary contribution. In the mother's womb this tiny fertilized egg rapidly grows and unfolds according to a systematic plan into a human baby that usually is born nine months later.

But even before birth there have been many important developments in the unborn infant which may have a great deal of influence on its later behavior. First, the heredity passed to the child from mother and father will ordinarily determine many of the physical characteristics of the child, for example, the color of its eyes, skin, and hair, its adult height, its sex, size of ears, nose, and other features.

It is much less certain how much influence heredity has on the behavior of people or on their intelligence. There are some rare and extreme cases in which the behavior or the limitation of intelligence is clearly due to heredity, but these are very unusual situations. But it is clear that what happens to a person during his or her life, especially in infancy and childhood, does indeed have a great deal of influence on that person's behavior and ability to function intelligently. It follows that the kind of care, attention, and experiences a child is given has a major role in the behavior patterns that the child develops.

Even while in the protective womb of the mother, the fetus is nonetheless subject to conditions that may result in considerable difficulties throughout its life. For instance, if the mother develops certain kinds of illnesses during pregnancy, such as measles, especially during the critical first three months of the embryo's development, the brain or other structures of the baby may not develop properly. The baby may be born with disabilities, some of which could be very severe. Similarly, if the mother does not eat an adequate and nutritious diet, the developing fetus may not receive the proper nutrition it needs to develop properly. Alcohol and drugs, and even certain medicines, that the mother takes go through the fetus' bloodstream and can have severely damaging effects. Other factors, such as physical injuries to the mother during pregnancy or during a difficult birth which might involve the infant's not receiving enough oxygen or receiving head damage in the process of being born, may limit the newborn.

Most of these difficulties, of course, can be avoided by the mother's taking good care of herself during pregnancy and seeking competent medical help for a difficult birth. Poor people are usually at greater risk for these kinds of early developmental and birth problems than are those who have better care facilities available. Still, most children are born without having had such disasters occur to them.

Stages of normal human development

This section very briefly summarizes the main features of the developmental stages of human life. Human development is an ongoing process from conception to death. Each stage of human development prepares the individual for the next stage and each stage is influenced by what has happened in earlier stages (Erikson, 1963).

Early infancy—birth to 1½ years

Human beings are born as very helpless, dependent creatures who require close physical care and attention. A human infant starts with very little control, coordination, or ability to do much more than cry, suck, and eliminate. It requires almost complete care. However, rapid developmental changes occur during this period. Toward the end of the period the initially helpless, uncoordinated creature is walking, beginning to talk, may have urinary and bowel control, and most usually has formed a close relationship with its mother and a beginning relationship, perhaps, with a few others. To survive, the infant must have its basic needs met. The infant's security and confidence perhaps set the tone for its basic trust in the world and others that it will carry with it throughout its life.

Later infancy—1½ to 3½ years

During this period the infant continues to grow rapidly. Control and coordination of its body increase and improve to a remarkable degree. Children of this age are very active, curious, and into everything. This is the time when the child has a great need and energy to explore and use its new walking and motility seemingly constantly. This usually has to be met with increasing restrictions and insistence on limitations for the child's own safety and for the parents' sanity. As the child begins to assert its independence it can be stubbornly resistant to demands and restrictions. The child now has a greatly increased vocabulary. It can communicate in words and understand more and more of the complicated speech of others. Although still very dependent on the mother or mother substitute, the child in this period is gaining increasing independence and increasing ability to get along on its own. Social relationships are less exclusively directed to the mother and increasingly include other family members. Learning to control and coordinate bodily functions and establishing independence and confidence in beginning to do things for itself are characteristic of this period. Failure to achieve this kind of independence and confidence may be a source of doubt and insecurity which the child may be burdened with for the rest of its life.

Early childhood—3½ to 6 years

In this period there are some important changes for the child. Physically, it continues to grow and to develop rapidly. Coordination and control over the body increase, as do the child's knowledge, understanding, and capacity for much new learning. Usually during this time the child increases its social awareness and develops relationships outside the immediate home, finding playmates in the neighborhood or in nursery school. The child's sexual identity as a male or as a female tends to become firm. The basic aspects of the child's conscience are formed during this period, and controls over the child's behavior begin to shift from the parents and influences outside the child to the child's own self-direction as to what it should and shouldn't do. At this time the child begins to develop its own standards and to some extent it can direct its own behavior accordingly. However, the child still has a long way to go before being really fully capable of self-direction and control. From this start, self-control and self-direction normally increase steadily and continuously, ideally throughout the person's life. As the child's ability to develop its own standards and direct its own behaviors increases and is used successfully, the more confidence the child will have in its own ability to start and direct its behavior to satisfy its own needs and interests. If these efforts at self-direction do not function well or if they meet with frustration and failure, the child may begin to feel inadequate or guilty and may carry that burden as it goes on in life.

Middle and late childhood—6 to 12 years

During this period the child generally seems ready and open for formal school learning. It is at this time that the child acquires the basic educational and technical skills needed for its particular society and particular culture. Furthermore, it is also a time for learning the social rules and behaviors of a culture. As a result of spending much time in school and by forming close attachments to other children of the same age and sex, the child is less often at and less involved in the home. Influences outside the home expand and may sometimes conflict with the values and standards of the home. This is a time of acquiring the work habits and patterns of the culture, of acquiring the tools needed to fit in to one's own society, and for developing social relationships with peers outside the home. Failure to do so may result in a continuing sense of inadequacy and failure and an inability to fit into society.

Adolescence—12 to 18–25 years

Adolescence is the period of change from childhood to adulthood. It is a period of physical growth, bodily changes, and physical maturity and of adult sexual development and intense sexual interest and striving. Psychologically, it is also a time of change, from childhood to adulthood and from dependence to independence. Importantly, it is a period for the individual to establish fully a sense of who and what he or she is and to find a direction in life. During this period, and as part of the process of finding oneself, it is also a time for establishing relationships with others socially, sexually, and competitively. For many individuals, adolescence may be a difficult period of upset, of rapidly changing moods and behaviors, and sometimes of highly conflicting states. The adolescent does much experimenting and testing of this new role, the new physical body, and the new physical needs. This is a period in which much personal growth and maturing occur, or failing that, a time of confusion. Failure to develop new modes of behavior may be the result of the adolescent's being unable to deal with the pressures and changes of the new social position and the demands and changes of his or her physical body.

Adulthood—from 20 to 25 years

Although the end of adolescence means the end of physical growth and the completion of full physical sexual development, people continue to mature and develop throughout life, and eventually change and decline. Adulthood can also be viewed in terms of definite developmental periods or phases. However, with adults, the phases may not be as similar from person to person nor as different from each other as are the earlier phases. In addition, the adult phases are not as clearly linked to definite ages and may overlap much more so than do the earlier developmental phases. We are only now beginning to study and understand more about the adult phases of life. Three phases of adulthood will be considered below.

Early adulthood

Establishing independence in emotional, social, and self-support areas as well as in living arrangements is the major task of the early adulthood period. Establishing full adult independence and social relationships is ideally based on full give and take and on sharing and caring for others. This is a time of finding relationships and partnerships with others which are based on mutual give and take and meeting each other's needs. These are relationships in terms of love, friendships, working colleagues and peers, and competition. Failure to establish such close, intimate sharing relations leads to a socially isolated lonely existence.

Middle adulthood

The middle adulthood phase is most characterized by the finding of a partner and pairing with another in love and closeness and in jointly producing and sharing children, a household, and developing a family. It is generally the time for establishing families, raising children, and developing a close, caring intimate partnership with another. However, the producing and sharing can be in terms of other things besides children, such as through artistic productions or through vocational development and efforts. Failure in some broad form to really create and develop things outside the self may result in a self-centered, self-concern orientation.

Later adulthood

Later adulthood is the period when the children are grown and leave home and when physical changes of decline begin to occur. These may be changes in strength and energy, in reproductive capacity, and for some, in speed and alertness. It can be a good time when adults are free from the responsibilities of raising children and can turn to the interests and pleasures which they had to give up while raising a family. There is a considerable change in role and freedom. Learning and knowing how to use free time and to enjoy interests beyond the responsibilities of raising a family are quite important. This can be a very pleasant and satisfying time of life for those who have learned such things or it can be an empty, boring time for those who have not.

Final phases of adulthood

Retirement from work and a gradual slowing of physical and mental vigor as well as more restricted social and family contacts may occur at this point. This can be a time of comfort and feeling of having done well at a job and having a sense of being of value to others for one's knowledge, experience, and wisdom. People who enter the final phase of life with such a view usually make a comfortable adjustment to the ultimate decline and the ultimate end. But for some, this period may be a time of feeling disappointment and failure. Such individuals may feel that they did not do all that they should have or could have, may feel that they have lost opportunities which now cannot be regained. Such people may come into the final period unhappy, disappointed, and fearful of death.

Each developmental phase is influenced by what has happened or has not happened in the phase that came before it. Difficulties in earlier phases complicate adjustment in later phases. The importance of giving children a good start from the very beginning cannot be overemphasized. But problems at any stage are, of course, unavoidable.

Each developmental phase presents certain challenges for new learning and adapting to new circumstances. This is the result of the person's developing or declining physical ability as well as the result of what his or her family, friends, society, and culture expect and of the way the person is treated. Furthermore, each individual must also adapt to the individual stresses and circumstances of his or her particular life situation.

Adapting and adjustment—coping with stress and frustration

At every period of life and in almost every situation people, in order to adjust, must solve problems, make choices, face disappointments and frustrations, and deal with stresses, pressures, and demands. For instance, even a newborn infant in its helplessness must and can let its needs to be fed be known. Equipped with a piercing cry that can become intense and demanding, the infant can and must bring forth gratification from the mother or mother substitute. This is one of the earliest examples of how people begin to learn to cope and satisfy their needs.

By age ten a child must deal with many more difficult problems. For instance, consider the problem faced by the boy whose teacher demands that he learn arithmetic and whose friends pressure him to be part of a group passing notes in class. The teacher has to deal with her anger and frustration at the child's inattention and with her need to keep her job so that she can support her family. Or a wife may have to deal with her husband's drinking and interest in other women. Or an older person may have to come to grips with the fact that she can no longer see well enough to do her own cooking or house cleaning.

Learning to cope and adjust to the stresses and frustrations of living starts at birth and is a lifelong process. In many ways it is a process of building capabilities to develop an effective means to handle stress. When pressures and stress are more than an individual can deal with adequately, *distress reactions* begin to show themselves. These reactions may take one of several forms: (1) A fearful panic or anxiety reaction whereby the individual feels tense, irritable, worried, and afraid, often with no clear idea of why. (2) An angry outburst and an attempt to directly attack or destroy what seems to be frustrating the individual. Patterns of hurting or destroying others or property or sometimes oneself result from this kind of response to stress. (3) Withdrawal into oneself, paying little attention to other people or other things, and trying to live in a world of one's own. (4) Turning to some substance, such as alcohol or other drug, to try to gain some feeling of well-being and escaping, at least temporarily, from the problem.

There seem to be certain conditions that more so than others increase the chances of an emotional disturbance. These are factors that increase stress on a person's adjusting capabilities. Some of the major ones are as follows: (1) The chances of an emotional breakdown are increased under conditions of stress for people who have been unable to learn how to successfully cope with problems. (2) It is possible that some people are born with a greater reactivity to stress and frustration than are others. Such persons may have more difficulty adjusting and may be more likely to have an emotional breakdown than others. (3) Physical and health handicaps increase the amount of stress and lower tolerance. (4) Malnutrition reduces the ability to adjust and may even cause permanent brain injury in young children. (5) Excessive fatigue and lack of sleep increase the vulnerability to stress.

Family factors and early life experiences also create distress reactions. (1) Children who are not given regular care, attention, and loving may experience much early frustration. Their ability to deal with stress may be lowered. Basic coping skills for later adjustment may then be considerably limited. Family patterns of children who are rejected, that is, not wanted or cared for, and sometimes even physically abused, also create distress reactions. The opposite of rejection, that is, overprotection and restrictiveness, can also have the serious effect of not permitting the child to experience and learn how to deal with normal frustrations and thus not gain the needed skills for coping with problems. Overpermissiveness and indulgence may also result in the child's failing to learn to control its impulsiveness and desires. The result may be a selfish, inconsiderate, and demanding person who is likely to find great frustrations later on. (2) Parents who behave in patterns of ineffectiveness or maladjustment present a model that well might influence the child's behavior toward the same poor adjustment.

Other severe stresses that can lead to overwhelming one's adjusting mechanisms are: (1) A major failure experience. (2) The loss of a very close relative or friend; sometimes for adults even loss of money or status has the same effect. (3) Lack of personal resources, such as education, job, or money which prevents the individual from being part of the rest of society, is important. (4) Factors such as guilt and loneliness are also important aspects of vulnerability. (5) The stresses of poverty, low economic status, and lack of employment can lead to feelings of uselessness and worthlessness. These feelings may reduce a person's ability to cope with other stresses.

Defense mechanisms

When people are faced with problems, conflicts, or other stresses, the initial response usually is anxiety which is experienced as discomfort or tension. Anxiety can be a very uncomfortable and painful feeling of distress and uneasiness or a sense of dread or fear. Often the person has no clear idea about the source of these feelings. Anxiety also has physical aspects which may include restlessness, inability to stay still or sleep well, or more rapid breathing and heartbeat, sweating, and raised blood pressure. Digestive and bowel distress is not uncommon. These obviously are very uncomfortable feelings from which the person tries to escape.

There is a wide range of behaviors which people are capable of in attempting to turn off their felt anxiety and distress. A *defense mechanism* is any behavior or thought process people use to protect themselves against very stressful or personally threatening circumstances in order to reduce the anxiety. When not overused and when they are part of a number of other ways of coping, defense mechanisms can be very helpful. We all use many of these mechanisms frequently and even routinely in our everyday behavior. It is only when they are used too often, too rigidly, or to the exclusion of other means, as happens in desperate efforts to deal with stress, that they become a poor, even maladaptive means of trying to cope. Under those circumstances, some defense mechanisms may cause as much or more adjustment difficulty for the individual than they solve.

Many defense mechanisms have been described, but some of the more common ones are considered below. It must be remembered that they often do overlap each other and seldom are they present without interacting with other defense mechanisms or coping strategies.

Repression

One common, and in some ways basic, defense mechanism is repression. The person attempts to block the awareness of what is upsetting, conflicting, or frustrating. Painful, threatening thoughts, urges, wishes, or experiences are pushed out of the person's awareness. Repression may reduce the discomfort and anxiety, but it does not change the problem or the stress, which usually continues to have its effect even though the individual who is repressing the source now has no clear idea what it is that is bothering him or her. It is important to note that repression, like other defense mechanisms, occurs automatically and is not a deliberate action on the person's part. Repression has sometimes been called *selective forgetting*. It is different from *suppression*, which is deliberately choosing not to express what one is aware of.

An example of repression is that of a man who while driving to work was involved in an automobile crash which killed the driver of the other car. The man in question was uninjured physically, but he had no memory of the accident at all. However, following the accident he began to experience extreme attacks of anxiety and panic, to sleep very poorly, and to experience very frightening nightmares. With the help of psychotherapy and hypnosis he was able to recall and to experience the extremely stressful, frightening, and guilt-laden emotions surrounding the accident (even though he was not at fault), as well as to recall his fright and fear at the time for his own life. Having brought the source of his anxiety to awareness, he was gradually able to come to terms with it.

Denial

Denial is in some ways similar to repression, but denial involves a person's denying what he or she sees, hears, thinks, or feels. It is as if they are not there at all or that a stressful situation just cannot be so. Basically, denial is a process of ignoring the existence of what is there. An example is that of a woman whose husband recently died. She nonetheless continued to prepare meals for him, to wash and iron his clothes, and plan her life as if he were still there.

Regression

Regression involves falling back on earlier patterns of behavior, usually of a more immature level, as a way to cope with conflict and anxiety. A child who was toilet trained and was speaking well began wetting again, talking baby talk, and having tantrums when a new baby arrived, thus taking its mother's time and attention. This is a not uncommon example of regression.

Reaction formation

Reaction formation is a process whereby the person's outward attitude is the opposite from the person's true feelings. For example, an individual who outwardly behaves in a very helpful, generous way may be reacting against underlying angry, destructive impulses. Another individual who becomes involved in a crusade against gambling may be defending against his or her own impulses to gamble. In reaction formation the outward behavior very often is overdone. The forbidden, real urges may nonetheless come through in their association with the behavior which is the opposite of the impulse. For instance, in a crusade against pornography, the crusader has to find and experience pornography in order to put a stop to it. In reaction formation the underlying feeling is never very far beneath the surface.

Projection

Projection is a prominent means of trying to avoid anxiety by unrealistically blaming other persons or situations for the urges, problems, or feelings which the individual cannot accept in himself or herself. Thus, one's own faults, failings, or forbidden wishes are seen in others rather than acknowledged as part of oneself. An example is that of a man who became interested in another woman who was not his wife. However, to protect himself against the guilt and conflict about this situation, he began to suspect and accuse his wife of being interested in or having affairs with other men. In another case, a man was very angry with his boss. Since this anger was unacceptable, the man experienced that his boss was angry with him and was trying to have him fired.

Isolation

In isolation different aspects of experience are kept separate from each other so that the meaning and impact of them are not experienced. Thus, one may talk about being very angry in certain situations but not feel the appropriate anger when doing so, or one may isolate his or her feelings of sadness at the death of a loved one and not experience sorrow at the funeral.

Intellectualization

Intellectualization is a means of isolating feelings by putting them at a detached distance through thinking and talking about things in very abstract and distant terms. A very adaptive use of intellectualization is the way a good surgeon can impersonally and scientifically cut a person open and remove parts. When excessively used to avoid facing one's feelings by always being involved in distant, abstract concerns, intellectualization can lead to problems in dealing realistically with one's own needs and life circumstances.

Rationalization

Through rationalization a person avoids the emotional stress of real feelings or situations by creating a possible but not true reason for his or her behavior. For instance, a young man asks a girl he is very interested in for a date. She turns him down. The young man rationalizes his hurt and disappointment by telling himself that she is a snob and he is glad that he found out before he went out with her.

Displacement

Displacement is a shifting of a feeling or a shifting of the person to whom the unacceptable feeling is directed to something or someone else. For example, a man who is frustrated and angry with his boss at work does not dare show it. When he goes home, however, he finds fault with his wife and displaces his anger to her and immediately starts an argument.

There are many more defense mechanisms and other means people use in attempting to cope with stress. Understanding that these are not deliberate behaviors and that the individual may well not be aware of using such methods can be useful to the clinician. Often therapy involves helping the individual recognize defense mechanisms and helping him or her to learn more effective and more realistic means of handling problems instead.

Major types of emotional and behavioral disorder

One major class of response to stress is that characterized by conflict and distress within the individual. The person with this disorder usually is experiencing much personal misery, anxiety, and very poor feelings about himself or herself. Although the person usually manages to somehow get by, the person lacks full effectiveness in dealing with life's circumstances. This reaction has been called *neurosis*. The new classification (American Psychiatric Association, 1980) considers most of these reactions to be either anxiety or dissociative disorders. Even though the neurotic individual is often personally miserable and not as effective in life as he or she could be, the neurotic person generally functions realistically in society. Usually, the neurotic person can hold a job, have a family, and maintain some level of social relationships.

A more serious poor adjustment response is characterized by considerable disorganization in a person's thinking and feeling, with the result that the person can no longer reason or behave realistically in many situations. Such people may even develop strange sensations, such as hearing or seeing things that aren't there, develop false ideas about being mistreated, or unrealistically believe that they are famous or great. Such disorders are the most severe kind and are called *psychoses*. Still another group of disorders are those in which the person's emotional feelings of sadness or seeming happiness become so extreme that they become unrealistic and sometimes life threatening. These are called *affective* or *mood disorders*. Most frequently these are in the form of sadness and severe depression; suicide sometimes becomes a serious danger. More rare is the mood disturbance called *mania* in which the individual is highly excited or reactive, restless and somewhat aggressively so, but in a context of being overly optimistic and merry. The individual is often frequently joking.

Personality disorders are behavioral difficulties which tend to be a characteristic style of behaving and reacting of long-standing. The individual with a personality disorder neither experiences much internal anxiety or distress nor is extremely unrealistic in his or her behavior. Nonetheless, the behavior pattern causes difficulty in that the person's ability to relate warmly and fully to others, the person's general effectiveness, socially and vocationally, are interfered with. Sometimes there is a pattern of social and legal difficulty.

There are some additional behavioral disorders which are clearly related to known brain damage due to such factors as head injuries, brain impairment as the result of deterioration with aging, or brain damage from drugs and alcohol. However, for most of the disorders, no known actual physical brain damage or hereditary basis has been fully established. It is assumed that for most disorders, experiences and the stresses of life are major factors in the disorders.

There are also still other forms in which maladaptive behaviors can occur. One is that of being unable to conform regularly to rules and laws of one's group, culture, and society. Delinquent children and some adult criminals fall into this category. Addiction to drugs (including alcohol), which is a poor attempt to cope with problems and stress, is also a very common disorder. In addition, there are many types of difficulties related to sexual behavior and performance. These have to do with an inadequate ability to perform or experience pleasure in sexuality or involve sexual gratification in ways in which society disapproves, such as peeking, exposing, or hurting others.

Classification of mental disorders

The various types and forms of emotional and behavioral disorders are classified according to *The Diagnostic and Statistical Manual III* of the American Psychiatric Association. This manual is also known as the *DSM III*. These classifications are the standard shorthand and way of designating and talking about different types of emotional disorders. Mental health workers must become familiar with these basic categories and terms.

In the *DSM III* each individual is evaluated in five categories: I. Clinical psychiatric syndrome (the familiar diagnostic category). II. According to any basic personality disorders. III. Including any physical disabilities or disorders. IV. Indications of the severity of environmental stresses or pressures. V. Indications of the highest level of adaptive functioning of that person during the previous year.

The major clinical psychiatric syndromes (Axis I) from the *DSM III* are briefly outlined below:

A. Disorders Usually First Evident in Infancy, Childhood, and Adolescence

> Mental Retardation
> Pervasive Developmental Disorders
> Specific Developmental Disorders (Axis II)
> Attentional Disorders
> Conduct Disorders
> Anxiety Disorders of Childhood and Adolescence
> Other Disorders of Infancy, Childhood, or Adolescence
> Eating Disorders
> Stereotyped Movement Disorders

B. Organic Mental Disorders

> Dementias
> Substance-induced (Drug-Alcohol)

C. Substance-use Disorders (Drug-Alcohol)

D. Schizophrenic Disorders

> Disorganized, Catatonic, Paranoid, Undifferentiated, Residual

E. Paranoid Disorders

F. Psychotic Disorders Not Elsewhere Classified

> Schizoaffective

G. Affective Disorders

H. Anxiety Disorders

I. Somatoform Disorders

J. Dissociative Disorders

K. Personality Disorders (Axis II)

L. Psychosexual Disorders
Gender Identity Disorders
Paraphilias
Sexual Dysfunctions

M. Factitious Disorders

N. Adjustment Disorders

O. Disorders of Impulse Control Not Elsewhere Classified

P. Psychological Factors Affecting Physical Condition

Q. Conditions Not Attributable to Mental Disorder

summary

1 Factors influencing the development of human behavior include hereditary potential, various nutritional, disease, injury, or drug factors while the child is still being carried by the mother, and injuries at birth.

2 People develop through orderly stages that are ongoing through life; each development builds upon previous developments.

3 Early infancy starts with helpless dependency, but in a year's time the child is walking, beginning to talk, and has formed a close relationship with the mother. Learning to trust the world is the positive outcome of this period. Later infancy is a time of curiosity, active intrusion, and exploration. The developmental task is independence, or failing that, doubt and insecurity.

4 Early childhood is a time for developing play relationships outside the home, establishing a sex role, and a conscience so that behavior is increasingly controlled by the child's own standards. Self-starting and self-direction are positive outcomes. Middle childhood is a time for school and for learning the basic skills of a culture. Establishing work habits to cope with the tasks of society is a positive result; a sense of abiding inferiority occurs when this fails.

5 Adolescence is the time of change from childhood to adulthood. Establishing a firm sense of oneself and one's direction is the major task of this period.

6 Psychological development continues throughout life. Early adulthood focuses on developing close intimate relationships, middle adulthood on sharing, caring, and generating new life and ideas, and later adulthood on accepting one's accomplishments and failures and enjoying the fruits of one's life endeavors.

7 At every stage of life people are faced with problems, conflicts, and frustrations with which they must cope. Factors from earlier developmental experiences and physical circumstances make some individuals more resistant to emotional disturbance than are others.

8 Defense mechanisms are behaviors people use to avoid painful anxiety and to protect themselves from emotional threat. Used moderately and in combination with other means, defense mechanisms are adaptive, but when they are used intensely and exclusively they may become a source of maladjustment. Some of the major defense mechanisms are repression, regression, denial, isolation, projection, and reaction formation.

9 Major emotional disorders are classified according to symptom patterns and behaviors. Neuroses or anxiety and dissociative reactions are characterized by internal discomfort and ineffectiveness in some aspect of a person's life, but the person has a basic hold on reality. Psychoses are much more disruptive and involve dangerous disturbances in ability to cope with reality. Other forms involve disturbances of mood and fixed patterns of poor effectiveness. The *DSM III* provides the standard classifications of emotional disorders.

Recognizing the signs and types of emotional disorder

Having a technical name such as neuroses or psychoses by itself isn't of much help to people with emotional problems. The mental health worker does, however, need to recognize the signs of the major classifications or types of disorder because they give the practitioner some idea of whether or not he or she is dealing with a serious, even life-threatening reaction, or mild one, or maybe behavior that is not really unusual at all. The kind of treatment needed or not needed, to some extent, is related to the type of disorder, and to some degree the correct knowledge of the disorder can give the mental health worker some idea about what to look for and to expect in in the behavior of certain individuals.

Furthermore, classifications of mental disorders are used by most mental health professionals, hospitals, and clinics. Familiarity with the terms and classifications will help the mental health worker communicate with these people and institutions. Most emotionally upset individuals, however, don't neatly fit into any one classification. The concern should not be with putting a label on a disturbed person but rather with considering how that person tries to cope and with how the person can be helped. A brief description of the major current classifications of disorder based on the *DSM III* follows.

Adjustment disorders

Given enough frustration or stress, anyone can experience an emotional disorder. Such things as terrifying accidents, sudden loss of loved ones, being fired from a job, being put in prison, long periods of not having enough food or water, military combat, among other such events can result in a temporary personality breakdown.

While the breakdown may take many forms, from feeling highly tense or irritable, anxious or depressed, to losing control or reality orientation, these situational difficulties usually improve rapidly when the person is removed from the stressful circumstances.

A *post-traumatic shock reaction* is a condition that may come on rather suddenly in response to stress. Sometimes, however, the reaction builds up slowly, as might be the case of a soldier who remains in a combat stress situation for a long period.

Most commonly the symptoms are those of anxiety which are sometimes accompanied by feelings of sadness, depression, fear, and tension. A tendency to *depersonalize,* that is, to feel that things are not quite real, is also a common reaction in situational disorders. It is as if one is watching oneself do things instead of being a real part of the situation.

Sometimes the initial reaction to a sudden major stress is that of a severe *shock reaction.* Here the person seems rather dazed and confused and may wander aimlessly. Even memory of the stressful event may be lost. As the shock stage passes, a suggestible stage often follows. The person in this stage tends to be passive, docile, and quite willing to follow orders from others. During this phase the individual frequently expresses much concern about the safety of others but is still very inefficient in being able to do even routine tasks. The person begins to experience tension and anxiety as he or she gradually begins to regain full psychological functioning.

Neuroses

The common feature of the group of disorders known as neuroses is that the individual experiences anxiety, personal dissatisfaction, and unhappiness and is usually ineffective and inefficient in at least some important areas of his or her life. The neuroses develop over a long period and tend to continue even when the person is not under any great stress. Despite these uncomfortable experiences, neurotics usually manage to maintain their jobs and function socially and within their families, but they do so with great difficulty and effort. Neurotics are aware that their behavior is inefficient and it even may seem strange to them. Thus, they are not impaired in their understanding of reality, although they are often unable to behave in more realistic ways.

In the *DSM III* classification these disorders are no longer grouped together under the term neuroses. They are now contained in the categories of *anxiety* and *dissociative disorders* and are included along with other disorders in the *affective, somatoform,* and *psychosexual disorders.*

Anxiety disorders

This category includes the anxiety states in which the primary symptom is an intense, uncomfortable sense of apprehension. This fear and tension is usually associated with physical symptoms of rapid heartbeat, increased blood pressure, rapid breathing, sweating, trembling, dizziness, and others.

In the *anxiety-panic disorder* there are recurrent sudden anxiety attacks of varying acute fears or terror associated with feelings of impending disaster. The panic experiences are very severe, although they usually do not last very long, but they recur repeatedly.

Generalized anxiety disorder is characterized by a persistent, continuous sense of uncomfortable anxiety that lasts over a period of at least one month. The same general symptoms of tension, anxiety, and fear and many of the physical types of the reactions are present, although not in the extreme form of panic reaction.

Phobic disorders involve continuous unrealistic fears of certain things, activities, or situations to such a degree that the individual feels great fear and attempts to avoid the feared thing. In *agoraphobia* the person is markedly afraid to be alone or in public places where escape is difficult or to be where help would not be easily available should he or she need it. For instance, being in a big crowd, or on a bridge, or in a tunnel.

Social phobia, which is also common, is an irrational fear and compelling desire to avoid situations in which a person might be observed by others. Fears of performing or speaking in public, eating in public, using public toilets, and so forth are included in this category.

Simple phobia refers to fears of very specific things. These phobias generally are not as incapacitating as the other forms of phobia. Some examples of these might be fears of specific animals such as dogs, cats, or insects, or of closed places, or of heights.

In *obsessive and compulsive disorders* the anxiety is focused and is thus not directly experienced. Rather, the person tries to avoid anxiety through obsessions which are persistent thoughts and ideas that seem to occur involuntarily and are thought to be senseless and often very undesirable. The obsessive person, however, cannot stop such thoughts. These thoughts may have to do with such things as committing immoral acts, attempting suicide, or be about the functions of his or her body.

Compulsions are repeated actions the individual feels compelled to carry out even though the actions may often seem strange and ridiculous to the individual. These might be such behaviors as avoiding stepping on cracks in the sidewalk, washing four times before every meal, making the sign of a cross before entering any building, or having to touch certain objects whenever they are viewed.

Dissociative disorders

The main feature of this group is that of temporary and often sudden change in awareness with regard to memory of personal events or in an individual's usual sense of identity. Who the person is may be forgotten temporarily and sometimes a new identity is assumed.

A psychologically based *amnesia reaction* is the sudden inability to remember important information about oneself; it goes much beyond just ordinary forgetting. In this case, the disturbance is not due to brain damage or alcohol blackouts.

The psychological *fugue state* is a somewhat more extreme form of forgetting and usually involves the individual's leaving his or her customary place of living and taking up a new identity while being able to recall his or her previous identity.

Multiple personality

Some individuals may develop several sometimes completely different and opposite personalities. The personalities may shift back and forth with each one having no awareness of the existence of the others. Each of the personalities has a distinct development with its distinct behavioral style and social relationships. A *depersonalization disorder* refers to a dissociative state in which an individual experiences a sense of unreality as if he or she were seeing himself or herself from a distance or as a spectator.

Somatoform disorders

In somatoform disorders the individual experiences or complains of physical symptoms, but there is no evidence of a known physical disorder. The symptoms are considered to be associated with psychological conflict. These disorders are not under voluntary control, and the individual is experiencing a physical difficulty.

Somatization disorders

Somatization disorders are characterized by continuing and multiple physical complaints of several years duration for which the individual has gone for medical help but for which there is no physical disorder found. The complaints are often dramatic but rather vague. In order to fit the category, there must be a number of physical symptoms which may include problems in functioning of different bodily organs, digestive complaints, pain, or symptoms having to do with breathing and the heart.

Conversion disorders

Conversion disorders involve a clear loss or change in functioning that suggests a physical disorder for which there is no physical basis. Typical conversion symptoms may involve blindness, deafness, loss of feeling to parts of the body, paralysis, or other such disorders. These disabilities usually do not conform to the physical makeup of the body. But the individual appears to experience anxiety reduction by focusing on the physical condition.

In the *psychogenic pain disorder* there is a complaint of severe prolonged pain, but it isn't consistent with the pain pathways of the body and there appears to be no organic basis for it, or if there is, the complaint of pain is greatly in excess of what would be expected.

Hypochondrais is an overexaggerated interpretation of bodily signs or sensations as being abnormal. The individual becomes constantly concerned with a fear or a belief that he or she has a very serious physical illness. There is no physical basis for the concern, but the individual is not reassured and in fact becomes socially or vocationally impaired.

Neurotic depression, now called *dysthymic disorder,* is classified under the affective disorders. It involves a long-standing depressed mood or loss of interest and sense of pleasure in most things in life for a period of several years. The person feels sad, low, and unhappy. There is no extensive disruption of social or vocational functioning. The individual may have insomnia, feel chronically tired, have a low sense of self-esteem, frequently cry, or have recurring thoughts of death or suicide.

Treatment of neuroses

There are several approaches that are useful in dealing with neurotic problems. The anxiety and tension can be helped by aiding the person to better deal with stressful situations and to learn how to relax and sometimes by tranquilizing pills. Counseling, either individual or group, may aid the individual to understand his or her behavior and develop new ways of dealing with situations. Behavioral methods aimed at specific symptoms like phobias and obsessional thoughts are also useful approaches.

Personality disorders

In personality disorders the individual has a long-standing pattern of behavior that reduces his or her effectiveness because of inflexible and maladaptive personality traits. In some instances, they result in acts which are not considered socially acceptable and may even be illegal. Many, but not all, delinquents and criminals would fall into the category of *antisocial personality disorder*. Such individuals do not ordinarily experience the intense anxiety and personal misery that the neurotics do. They well understand what socially acceptable behavior is, but they have little desire to conform or to behave differently.

These individuals tend to be impulsive, to be quite self-centered, and appear to have a relatively weak conscience and little concern for others. Some have considerable social charm and skill that they use to manipulate or gain advantage over others to satisfy their own wants.

Some other forms of personality disorder include the *paranoid personality disorder* characterized by an unwarranted, resistant mistrust and suspicion, an oversensitivity, and very restricted emotional expression. A *schizoid personality* is characterized by emotional coldness, indifference, fear of criticism, and few close friendships. The *histrionic personality* is overly dramatic, reactive, self-indulgent, shallow in relationships, and attention-seeking. The *passive-aggressive personality* resists demands for adequate social and job performance and through stubbornness, procrastinating, or forgetting.

Treatment of personality disorders

These behavior patterns and trait disorders are often very fixed and difficult to change. No one treatment method has been very successful with them. Environmental changes and behavioral therapies seem the most promising right now.

The addictions: Alcohol and drugs

Alcoholics become dependent both psychologically and physiologically on the drug alcohol for their sense of well-being. Drinking, or even getting drunk, is not the same as alcoholism, but alcoholics do both to excess. A person is considered an alcoholic when his or her drinking results in interference with any of the major aspects of his or her life. This could include disturbance of the family relationships with the spouse, children, or parents, disruption in functioning at work, harming health, or difficulty with the law.

There are many patterns of drinking and types of alcoholics. Some follow the long course of continually increased drinking with greater and greater behavioral and physical dependency and harm; other patterns of alcoholism consist of episodes of drunkenness with periods of sobriety in between.

Alcohol is the drug most frequently involved in addictions, but there are many other drugs and substances to which people also become addicted. Although not all of them are physically addicting, people can become psychologically dependent in a true addictive sense to a wide variety of substances.

There is no clear evidence of a particular type of person or personality who becomes addicted, but people who are addicted often have some similar behaviors such as dependency, unreliability, self-centeredness, and impulsiveness. Much of this could be the result of the addiction instead of the cause.

Because addiction, especially alcohol addiction, is so widespread, this is a disorder category of some importance.

Treatment of addictions

Treatment programs for addictions are available from a variety of standpoints. Most involve first drying out or getting the offending addictive substance out of the physical system of the addicted person and then working on the environmental and psychological stresses of the individual as well as helping develop less destructive means of gaining esteem and feelings of effectiveness. An extensive look at alcoholism is presented in Chapter 9.

Psychosexual disorders

Psychosexual dysfunctions

Psychosexual disorders have to do with the impairment of the desire for sex or the inability to achieve sexual gratification.

Male impotency This dysfunction refers to the inability of the male to gain or to maintain an erection. In primary impotence a male has never been successful in attaining an erection long enough to have successful sexual relations; in secondary impotence he has had at least some successful experience but is unable to maintain the erection. It is estimated that over half the male population on at least a temporary basis have suffered from secondary impotence.

Male ejaculatory incompetency This may consist of either premature ejaculation in which the male is unable to hold back long enough for his partner to achieve satisfaction or retarded ejaculation in which the male is unable to achieve the ejaculation. Considering all factors, the situations are those in which the male does not have voluntary control over his ejaculation. These are both fairly common forms of male sexual inadequacy.

Female orgasmic dysfunction In the primary form, sometimes referred to as *frigidity,* the female is essentially unable to experience sexual feelings and does not respond erotically to sexual stimulation. *Situational orgasmic dysfunction* refers to the inability of the female to achieve orgasm except in some very particular circumstances. Frigidity is relatively rare, but difficulties in achieving orgasm are a very common sexual complaint of women.

Vaginismus This refers to involuntary spasms of the muscles at the entrance of the woman's vagina which prevent penetration by the male and intercourse. It may occur either in a woman who is also frigid or in a woman who is otherwise aroused. Vaginismus is a relatively rare form of disorder.

Dyspareunia   In dyspareunia pain is experienced during sexual inter-course by either male or female.

Treatment of psychosexual dysfunctions

Sexual inadequacies are very often based in the person's attitudes, inhibitions, and guilt with regard to sexuality. These inadequacies are amenable to change by psychotherapy. Recently techniques have been developed using behavioral conditioning methods which have often provided considerable improvement and cures for these disorders. The methods for treating sexual inadequacy have proved very effective.

Nonadaptive and socially disapproved sexuality—Paraphilias

These disorders refer to sexual behavior which is considered socially offensive or dangerous and which is usually illegal.

Exhibitionism   In exhibitionism the person intentionally displays the sex organs to members of the opposite sex under inappropriate circum-stances. Most of the offenders are young adult males, although females can also be exhibitionists.

Voyeurism   A voyeur receives sexual pleasure through secret peeping, usually at members of the opposite sex who are undressing. Males are most often the offenders.

Fetishism   In fetishism the focus of sexual interest is on a certain part of the body or an outside object rather than the sexual organs. It most often occurs in males and the arousal objects can include such things as breasts, hair, ears, underclothing, shoes, stockings, and so forth. Such an individual may commit burglaries to steal the fetish object and usually masturbates when he has it in his possession.

Sadism   Sadists receive sexual stimulation and pleasure by inflicting pain on their sexual partners.

Sexual masochism   Sexual masochists become sexually aroused and receive pleasure from receiving pain and injury.

Incest   Incest is sexual intercourse between close relatives. Father-daughter sexual relationships are probably more frequent than mother-son relationships, which tend to be relatively rare. Brother-sister sexual relations are another form of incest. Considerable emotional damage and distress may result from these relationships, particularly to the child involved.

Pedophilia Pedophiliacs become sexually aroused and involved with children. Girls are more frequently the victims. Even young infants have been sexually molested by pedophiliacs.

Rape Rape is the crime of forcing an unwilling partner to have sexual intercourse. Statutory rape involves an individual who is under the legal age to consent. Legally it is considered rape even though the partner is very willing. Forcible rapes are often accompanied by a good deal of violence, and in many cases, hurting and humiliating the partner seem to be more the basis than the sexual gratification. Homosexual rapes can and do occur.

Treatment of socially disapproved sexuality

Psychotherapy and behavioral conditioning methods have been used with some effectiveness.

Alternative sexual patterns

There are other forms of sexuality that provide individuals with gratification. Some of them may be illegal. Nevertheless, they are becoming recognized as tolerable for consenting adults if no one is harmed.

Masturbation Masturbation is self-stimulation of the sex organs for gratification. Although it has been traditionally condemned on religious grounds, there are no known physical harmful effects. Masturbation is considered a normal, healthy outlet for young people and for people who are in situations in which other forms of sexual gratification are not available. The main undesirable feature of it is the worry and guilt and the self-devaluation that people may feel if they believe it is wrong.

Prostitution Prostitutes provide sexual gratification to others for a fee. Prostitution has been called the world's oldest profession. Again, while frowned on by religions and moral attitudes, it does provide gratification when other sexual outlets are unavailable. Prostitution most frequently involves a female prostitute and a male, but the reverse is also found—a male prostitute and a female. In addition, there are both male and female homosexual prostitutes.

Homosexuality   In homosexuality sexual attraction and behavior are directed toward an individual's own sex rather than toward the opposite sex. *Lesbianism* is the term for female homosexual relations. Homosexuality has been known throughout the history of mankind. It appears that those who are exclusively homosexual consist of two or three percent of the population, but a great many more individuals are *bisexual*, that is, are sexually aroused and gratified by both homosexual and heterosexual means. Furthermore, a great many people have experienced homosexual acts but have not continued in the orientation.

Evidence has revealed that most homosexuals generally function in normal average ways in society. There is probably no greater danger of homosexuals molesting young children than there is of pedophiliacs doing the same thing. Homosexuality as such is not now considered a form of psychopathology.

Transsexualism   A transvestite basically feels that he or she is a person of the opposite sex who has been trapped in the body of the sex he or she does not wish to be.

New surgical and medical techniques have made it possible to change the sex organs and hormones of such individuals so that they can become physically much like the sex they wish. For a male who wishes to become a female, the male organs are removed and replaced with an artificial vagina, and injections of female sex hormones are given which stimulate breast growth and development. In the case of females desiring to be male, the breasts, ovaries, and vagina are removed and a penis constructed from cartilage or plastic is attached to the body.

Affective disorders (disorders of mood)

While a disturbance of affect or mood frequently accompanies many forms of emotional disturbance, an affective disorder is characterized by the mood disturbance as the major symptom.

There are, of course, normal fluctuations in people's feelings of happiness or sadness and these mainly depend on the realistic situation a person is in. Thus, depression and sadness are appropriate at the loss of a loved one, and a feeling of happiness and excitement is appropriate at the point of achieving a great success or obtaining something that one has wanted very badly.

The affect disturbances become clinical problems when they persist beyond the reality of the situation. Remaining depressed years after one's mother's death or experiencing great sadness for no apparent realistic cause might be examples.

Depression

Mild depressions are characterized by feelings of sadness, discouragement, guilt, and low self-esteem and sometimes by irritability and restlessness. Sleep disturbance may also occur in depressions.

More *severe and profound depressions* can involve a lack of energy and ability to put forth effort that goes beyond slowing a person down. Sometimes the depression reaches the point that the person is in an acute immobilizing stupor. Feelings of self-unworthiness can become unrealistically and bizarrely extreme. In the *psychotic depression* the individual may have the unrealistic belief that he or she is the world's worst sinner, that he or she is so bad he or she doesn't deserve to eat, or that the body is so bad it is dead and rotting away.

In depressions there are very often thoughts of suicide and suicide attempts usually occur in individuals who are depressed. However, not all depressed individuals are suicidal by any means. But the risk of suicide in any given case must always be evaluated carefully when there are considerable symptoms of depression. Crisis therapy and suicide prevention are covered in Chapter 7.

Mania

Mania is an affective disorder in which there is an elevated mood of seeming excitement, gaiety, and joking and an expansive overly optimistic view of things. Such individuals tend to be very overactive, seem to have an overabundance of energy, and need little sleep. They talk rapidly and excitedly, and they take on too many tasks and commitments. In a fully developed manic excitement, such individuals may behave in a frenzied excitement of acitivity and shouting.

Treatment of affective disorders

Treatment for the milder forms of affective disorders involves helping individuals to become more active and involved in satisfying life activities, aiding them to understand the sources of their feelings, and aiding them to develop more satisfactory relationships and behaviors. In the extreme forms of affective disorder, patients sometimes must be hospitalized for their own protection. Suicide and suicide attempts occur in the context of depression and must always be seriously considered and evaluated in instances of severe depression.

Today there are psychotropic drugs which in some cases can be very effective against depressions and severe manic behavior.

Schizophrenia

Schizophrenia is probably the most frequent of the major psychotic reactions, that is, those severe disorders in which a person's ability to behave rationally and logically is severely impaired.

In general, schizophrenia is characterized by a disorder of thinking in which logic and reality of thought are usually very impaired. Schizophrenics sometimes show emotional responses that are inappropriate to the setting or situation which they are in. In addition, they often withdraw from social relationships and from involvements with their environment. This withdrawal is frequently associated with a substituted fantasy set of beliefs or relationships to which the schizophrenic reacts as if they were real. Schizophrenics often experience *hallucinations*, which are experiences of sights or sounds or feelings that have no basis in reality. Thus, a schizophrenic may hear voices calling him or her names, or see people or things which no one else can, or feel sensations that have no physical basis. To the schizophrenic, however, these are real and the schizophrenic responds to them.

Delusions are false beliefs, which sometimes are very elaborate. These can take several forms. A *persecutory delusion* is a false belief that someone or something is out to hurt or harm the individual. A *grandiose delusion* is a false belief that the individual has enormous powers or is in fact some famous person such as a king or God. A *delusion of reference* is the false belief that others are talking about the person or that news articles or TV shows are about that person. A *delusion of influence* is the false belief that one is being controlled or directed against one's will by outside forces, for example, rays or wires.

Paranoid schizophrenics are particularly characterized by their delusions or false beliefs.

In *catatonic schizophrenia* the individual may at some time go into a physical state of very tense, fixed body position and is unresponsive to anything around him or her. This state may alter with a wild angry period of excitement and physical assaults.

Disorganized-type schizophrenics tend to be particularly confused, inconsistent, and sometimes silly, and they behave in a very immature, primitive manner.

Treatment of schizophrenia

Schizophrenia either may occur in episodes in which the individual comes out of the disorder for varying periods of time or it may be continuous and progressive.

Supportive treatment, helping relationships, and assistance in dealing realistically with situations have been useful. Today there are effective drugs that counteract the most unusual and unrealistic behavior of these individuals. These drugs aid the individual to function without the severe symptoms of the disorder, but the drugs in and of themselves do not provide a basic change in the condition.

Organic brain disorders

There are some disorders in which impairment or damage to the brain is known to be the basic cause. The general symptoms found in conditions involving brain disorder usually include confusion, disorientation, irritability, difficulty in maintaining attention, and memory disturbances.

Drugs and alcohol affect the brain, and in the case of prolonged usage, they also destroy or injure portions of the brain. Drunkenness or various drug-induced states are a form of temporary brain disability, but extensive use can lead to permanent brain disability.

Diseases that attack the brain or cause high fevers can also result in organic brain symptoms. In addition, states of delirium occur under these conditions. Delirium in some ways is similar to the delusions and hallucinations of schizophrenia, but it usually is less well organized and is temporary.

Syphilis can eventually attack the brain and it is one of the diseases that may result in organic psychoses. Other physical states, such as extreme fatigue and chronic malnutrition or hunger, also have an effect on the brain and can result in organic-like behavior.

Actual brain damage may be the result of an accident or injury and may produce the symptoms discussed in this section. In addition, organic brain syndrome is found to be associated with old age in some cases. It is the result of a reduced supply of blood to the brain, or senile deterioration, conditions which become increasingly severe for some, but not all people, as they grow older.

Treatment of organic brain disorders

Treatment depends on whether or not the conditions are reversible. If there has been permanent destruction of part of the brain, the situation is less hopeful. Some drug and alcohol states improve dramatically when the drug or alcohol is out of the system, although extensive use of these substances can permanently damage the brain. Similarly, when fevers are reduced, provided that they haven't caused permanent damage, a good recovery should occur. When actual brain damage has occurred, the damaged portions of the brain cannot be replaced. In many instances, however, the individual can be trained to use other portions of the brain and improvement may occur.

Mental retardation

A little over two percent of the population is classified as mentally retarded. All but a small percentage of this two percent fall into the category of *mildly retarded*. Mildly retarded individuals develop intellectually at a slower rate than the rest of the population and they may only reach a peak level of learning that is comparable to a sixth- or seventh-grade individual. Such persons are, however, capable of getting along in the community, holding many kinds of jobs, and being productive members of society. But since they are limited in their understanding and ability, they may get into difficulty and can also be easily led and influenced by others. Hence, they may present something of a social problem. Many of these individuals do get into legal difficulty and spend time in prisons.

There is much uncertainty about the cause of mild retardation. Whether it is due to poor early environment or a lack of either stimulation, adequate nutrition, or early learning and training is not known. It well may be that most of these individuals, for the reasons cited, may have never had a proper opportunity to maximize their abilities.

The other categories of retardation are moderate, severe, and profound. They represent increasing levels of impairment. Many of these individuals also have physical handicaps, including brain damage and other bodily malfunctions. The higher functioning level individuals can be trained to provide self-help and care but they usually require supervision. The most severe of these cases may have to be institutionalized.

Treatment of mental retardation

Most retarded individuals can be educated or trained to function adequately and live successfully in the community, but they need supervision.

Disorders in children

Children grow and develop very rapidly and they almost constantly need to be making new adjustments to their expanding capabilities and the expanding environmental demands and pressures upon them. Many of the behavior disorders are brief and temporary and almost always are related to the developmental phase in which the child is in.

Some of the common problems include *problems in eating*. The main problems to be noted here are those of overeating because it results in *obesity*, which has both physical and psychological components, and *anorexia nervosa*, a pattern most often seen in adolescent girls who experience a loss of appetite, have an aversion to food, and lose extreme amounts of weight. Individuals can and have literally starved themselves to death.

Problems in toilet training include *enuresis* in which the individual has not gained control of passing urine at an age when other children have such control. Enuresis is more common during sleep but some individuals even at older ages may not have gained control during the daytime. There are a number of reliable and effective treatments for this.

Encopresis refers to the inability to control bowel movements. It is much less common than enuresis and there are methods for treating it.

Sleep disturbances, which may involve nightmares or sleepwalking, are common in children. The disturbance is usually related to an emotional stress or upset. Helping the child overcome his or her fears and anxieties will often resolve the problem.

Speech problems, including indistinct speech, baby talk, stuttering, or the inability to find the right words, occur and need to be treated in order for the child to be effective and secure.

Temper tantrums and *cruelty*, when extreme and repetitive, are often found with hyperactive attention disorders or with conduct disorders.

Learning disorders show themselves when the child is in school. They involve a variety of factors and call for careful assessment. The level of ability, the motivation to learn, and the capacity to hear and see should all be considered. These children are not retarded; they have specific impairments that interfere with learning.

Conduct disorders

Delinquency or committing acts that get the individual in trouble with the law is another major category of child disorder, especially toward the adolescent age range. Delinquency can have many causes that must be investigated.

Anxiety or *phobic reactions* in very frightened children seem to be related to insecurity. *School phobia,* or a refusal to go to school, is one of the more common aspects of this.

The *withdrawn child* who gets into trouble may be pressed or may have a much more serious problem than the boisterous child who gets into trouble. There are severe emotional withdrawal reactions in children which are much like schizophrenia in adulthood. *They are considered to be pervasive developmental disorders.* Early *infantile autism* and *childhood schizophrenia,* while rare, are such conditions.

A *hyperactive* child has symptoms of irritability, poor attention, distractibility, and poor learning. A minimal brain syndrome or a minimal damage to the brain has been suggested as a possible cause for this condition.

Treatment of disorders in children

A variety of treatment methods have proven effective for children. These are very specialized in each case. Behavior modification methods have been widely applied.

Psychological factors affecting physical condition

In these disorders bodily parts and functions are clearly affected and are at least partially the result of emotional factors. They differ from the conversion reactions in that actual physical structure or functioning is disabled. Stomach ulcers, high blood pressure, certain skin rashes, and asthma are examples of how nervous, tense, emotional states may affect the body and cause actual disorders. Treatment is often both medical and psychological.

summary

1 Mental health workers must be able to recognize the behaviors associated with the major types of emotional disorder. The classifications of disorders give some indication of the seriousness and type of treatment needed. Classification is also useful in communicating about cases.

2 Adjustment and post-traumatic shock reactions are temporary responses to severe stress. The symptoms are anxiety, depression, fears, and tension.

3 Neurosis manifests itself in continuous anxiety or defensive behavior to avoid anxiety that is relatively long lasting, experienced as uncomfortable, and is unacceptable to the neurotic, although the individual is unable to alter his or her behavior. The neurotic can usually function and be realistic. The neuroses include anxiety disorders, phobic disorders, obsessive-compulsive disorders, dissociative disorders, somatoform disorders, and neurotic depression.

4 Personality disorders are long-standing behavioral patterns that cause the person to be ineffectual or to get into trouble with society. They include the antisocial personality who frequently is in trouble with the law, the paranoid personality who is suspicious and guarded, the schizoid who is withdrawn and sometimes peculiar in behavior, and the histrionic who is very dramatic and attention seeking.

5 Drug and alcohol addictions and psychosexual disabilities represent other large categories of disturbance.

6 The affective disorders are characterized by an intense degree of mood domination of behavior, such as severe depression, or excited, overexpansive manic patterns.

7 Schizophrenia is the most prevalent and severe of the emotional disorders. It is a psychosis in which the individual's ability to deal realistically with his or her environment is severely impaired and in which hallucinations or delusions are often found. The general types of schizophrenia are paranoid, catatonic, and disorganized.

8 There are disorders resulting from brain damage. Memory loss and confusion are the most usual signs of brain damage.

9 Mental retardation refers to limited intellectual ability and is first noticeable in childhood. The levels of retardation range from mild to very profound disability.

10 Disorders of childhood vary in quality and extent from those of adults. They include eating, sleeping, and learning disorders, hyperactivity and interference with attention, anxiety withdrawal, and psychotic impairment of reality.

Part II

Clinical Methods and Techniques

Part 2 covers the basic methods and techniques that a practitioner in the mental health field is likely to find useful for a wide variety of clinical situations. In most cases, these basic methods also form the basis for many of the other more specialized methods that the practitioner will no doubt add to his or her skills as he or she continues in the field.

Interviewing, the subject of Chapter 6, is basic to almost all mental health situations. Although it may seem deceptively simple, the effective clinical interview requires a great deal of skill, practice, and understanding of the implications of what is being done.

Crisis intervention and *suicide prevention,* discussed in Chapter 7, are methods of treatment for acute situations, including suicidal behavior, requiring immediate attention. The methods and skills needed here will frequently be put to use by mental health practitioners.

Marital and family treatment methods, the subject of Chapter 8, are specialized approaches to these relationships and interpersonal problem situations. Counseling often involves couples or entire families and it involves dealing with group interactions.

Problem drinking and alcoholism and related problems are very frequently involved in the cases brought to the attention of the mental health practitioner. Knowledge of the disorder, its effects, and methods of treatment are covered in Chapter 9.

Several *special intervention methods* that may be of wide use to the mental health practitioner are touched on briefly in Chapter 10. The *behavior therapy* approach in general, *assertive training* specifically, *psychotropic medications,* and *sex therapy* are included. The *role of the patient advocate and how the social-welfare system works* are also covered.

Finally, in Chapter 11, the methods of prevention of emotional disorders and approaches to evaluating the effectiveness of intervention methods are covered.

Clinical Interviewing

6

Interviewing: The basic clinical tool

The interview is the major way in which helpers in the mental health profession come to understand the people with whom they are working, and specialized forms of interview are very frequently the main means of treating patients. Interviews are used for very many purposes in this field, and there are many forms of interviews as well as many styles of interviewing. The problems of the patient and the goal of the interview determine the form of the interview.

In some respects, something like interviewing is a natural part of the everyday way in which people interact and communicate in their normal living arrangements. It might then seem that no special training or skill is needed in order to be an effective clinical interviewer. After all, almost everybody knows how to talk to somebody else—or do they really?

It is very true that people at every social level and from every culture begin life in family groups and are very closely involved in the social interaction of their basic family. Right at birth the baby can let its wants be known by its crying, and the mother communicates a response to the baby by her actions and gestures. As speech develops, people communicate more and more with sounds and talk, but communication involves more than just talk. Actions and gestures, and what is called body language, are important in communication, as are the feelings and emotional expressions that accompany the words and actions. Since learning to communicate with others in these ways has been going on since birth, and since people have been practicing for many years, most people are reasonably good at social communication and with social interviews.

Clinical interviews depend heavily on the skills of social communication that people have developed in their lifetimes. Although clinical interviews and clinical interviewing have many similarities with social communication, in some very important ways they are distinct and different from social interviews.

Difference between clinical interviewing and social talking

While in some ways very similar, the clinical interview is basically different from the social interaction or conversation in a number of respects. Both the clinical interview and social conversation involve people talking together with the exchange of ideas, feelings, attitudes, and information. But social discussion and exchanges usually are not planned, and so have no set direction. In contrast, the clinical interview has been purposely arranged and has a definite direction and purpose, which give the clinical interview a focus and continuity around a particular set of problems or issues. Furthermore, in order for the clinical interview to achieve its purpose, one person must maintain the direction of the communication and keep it focused on obtaining the goal. This person is the interviewer.

Social discussions most usually are mutual and can and do go in any direction. In the clinical interview the direction and focus must be kept going toward its goal because the purpose of the clinical interview is to benefit the patient being interviewed. Generally, in such circumstances, the person being interviewed tells a great deal about the intimate details of his or her situation and life but the interviewer usually gives little information about himself or herself. Rather, the interviewer limits personal disclosures to professional activities. In a social discussion the parties interact with each other in an unplanned way. In a clinical interview the interviewer should have a clear plan and purpose for his or her actions, questions, and responses. The participants in the interview do not just happen to meet; the interview is planned for a definite time and place and the interview usually lasts a definite period of time. The clinical interview requires the full attention of the clinical interviewer. The interviewer cannot be casual and offhand in dealing with the person being interviewed, as can happen socially. Another important difference between social interaction and the clinical interview is that the clinical interview usually requires consideration of very un-pleasant information and feelings and social interactions usually do not.

The interviewer's training has taught the interviewer to understand the other person's personal difficulties usually much more completely than would be the case in most social interactions. This training has also provided the interviewer with methods for communicating this understanding. The professional interview is not a *mutual give-and-take social relationship*. Instead, it is a relationship in which the concern for, needs of, and welfare of the patient come first and the interviewer does not expect or ask for consideration of or interest in his or her needs and problems in return. The clinical interviewer does not bring his or her own problems into the relationship. In addition, the interviewer ordi-narily accepts what the other person communicates without responding with anger or with criticism. The decision about continuing the rela-tionship is not on the basis of how pleasant the other person's company might be. Also, the professional interviewer protects the time for the interview from interruptions and devotes full attention to the person being interviewed. Usually, the professional interviewer does not in-teract with the person being interviewed in other more social situations, although there are exceptions to this.

It should be clear from the above that the clinical interview and the role of the clinical interviewer are in many basic ways very different from ordinary social interaction situations and from social conversa-tions. The clinical interview has a definite purpose and the interviewer directs the interview toward achieving that purpose. Revealing infor-mation, feelings, and problems is largely the role of the one being interviewed; understanding these things, facilitating the communica-tion, and letting the person know that what has been said is understood is the role of the clinical interviewer. This requires much skill. The interviewer has the responsibility for arranging the time for the inter-view, for protecting the interview from interruptions, and for maintain-ing confidentiality of the material, and, ordinarily, the interviewer does not engage in social relationships with the patient, at least while the professional relationship is ongoing.

Types and purposes of the clinical interview

Interviews are used for a wide variety of nonclinical purposes and include employment interviews, interviews for newspapers and tele-vision, or interviews to gather research data, to name a few. The clinical interview is distinguished by its basic purpose: that of helping the client with regard to a personal and emotional problem situation. There are three general types of clinical interview: the assessment interview, the therapy treatment interview, and the consultation interview. Good clinical practice most often dictates that these interviews do not occur in separate distinct forms. For instance, therapy most often should be gradually begun even as the evaluation phase is ongoing. But, obviously, some evaluation is necessary in order to determine the type of appropriate therapy and its goals. The therapy interview must always be concerned with assessment and evaluation of where the patient is in order to determine how to proceed at any given time.

Assessment interview

The evaluation, assessment, or diagnostic interview has as its main goal and focus the assessment of the patient's problem in a full enough manner that the appropriate and effective intervention techniques may be employed. For an adequate assessment of this kind, it is necessary that the interviewer develop certain kinds of information on the patient and the patient's situation and that the interviewer accurately observe the patient's behavior and responses. As noted previously, for various reasons it is often important to commence therapy even while assessing the patient. One reason may be that the patient is under so much stress that some reduction of the symptoms and some sign that help is forthcoming are important. Even when the stress is not of an immediate crisis nature, giving the patient a beginning therapy experience can be a good start later toward quicker, more efficient therapy.

   Although it is useful, especially for an experienced interviewer, to have a standard set of areas of information to cover or even standard questions to ask, a much better relationship and atmosphere for the interview are created when the topics are covered as they become relevant to the patient's expressions of problems, rather than to try to cover them in a rigidly systematic way regardless of what particular aspect of the problem the patient is concerned about. There are some generally important areas that ordinarily should be included for an adequate assessment of the patient. These areas are listed below (see also Evaluation Interview Report on pages 90–91) in order of convenience. It is not necessary to follow the sequence.

Identifying information

From the standpoint of clinic or hospital records, for purposes of billing or knowing how to contact the patient or the family, and in order to know something of the individual's living situation, the following information should be obtained: the patient's name, address, and phone number, the date of birth, the date and place of the interview, the patient's housing and family situation, the name and address of the nearest relative or friend who can be contacted, the patient's educational level, occupation, marital status, number of children, the previous history of health or mental difficulties, and ethnic cultural background. Of course, other similar information may be helpful in a given case.

Reason for referral and referral source

The referral source, whether it is a self-referral or from an outside source, such as the family doctor, the court, or a friend, should be noted. The statement of the problem as seen by the outside source should also be obtained.

Patient's statement and view of the problem

It is very important to carefully and fully understand how the patient sees and feels about his or her problems and difficulties. It would not be unusual for the patient to view his or her situation in a very different way from that of the referral source. How the patient sees the problem also often gives many clues to how to work with and help the patient. It says something about the patient's motivation for help and also what it is that the patient is prepared to work on.

Information about the problem from other sources

It is often very helpful to obtain information about the problem from sources other than the patient. Although this isn't always necessary or possible, often it can add much to the understanding of the case, especially when dealing with children. For instance, in the case example on pages 93–95 what the teacher and the principal have to say provides important additional information about the child's situation in school. Some other sources of information may be obtained from police, courts, other clinics, relatives, and friends.

Behavior and description of the patient during interview

The assessment interview provides an opportunity to observe various important aspects of the patient's behavior and capabilities. A description of the patient's appearance, dress, and manner can be important. How the patient relates to the interviewer is useful information. Is, for instance, the patient reluctant and withholding, responding only minimally to questions, or very cooperative, open, and responsive? What are the mood and feelings expressed by the patient and how appropriate are they? Is the patient's logic and thinking clear? How is the patient's memory? Does the patient seem cold and indifferent, very sad and depressed, or unconcerned? How intelligent does the patient seem to be? How well can the patient express himself or herself in words or by other means? Does he or she seem anxious and under stress or is he or she bland or indifferent?

Precipitating factors and the patient's immediate situation

There are almost always events in the patient's immediate situation that have led to the patient's being referred or to coming in to seek help. These precipitating factors should be determined. The assessment interview should not only give a picture of the patient's immediate life situation, including the family living arrangements, significant relationships, jobs, finances, and other areas of importance, but also determine any change in status in the patient's life that may have triggered the disorder. A financial or employment reversal or a change in relationship with an important person are factors that should be explored.

Social and developmental history

A detailed social and/or developmental history may or may not be important and useful. It depends on the problem and case. In many cases, the problem and the focus of treatment will be on situations in the current life environment of the individual and a great deal of stress on the past background will not add much to the patient's treatment. There are, however, cases in which occurrences in earlier stages of the patient's life are crucial to the current problem and treatment. Here it is important to have a history of the individual's development and social interactions.

For example, in dealing with a child suspected of being retarded or having organic brain damage, information on the child's birth and early physical development, nutrition, illnesses, and so forth can be very helpful. Equally useful is information on the earliest relationships with the mother and father, siblings, friends, family, and so forth. Knowledge of an individual's response to schooling, to friends, and to dating and of an individual's sexual attitudes and experience may all add greatly to understanding a particular case and promoting treatment.

Medical history

The patient's current state of health, past serious illnesses and injuries, and the kinds of medicine the person is taking can be important factors in understanding the person and should be considered as part of the overall evaluation. Consulting with a physician about these matters may be necessary.

Assessment formulation of the problem

The information the interviewer obtains from the assessment interview is used to assess the nature of the individual's difficulty, to assess the individual's strengths and weaknesses for dealing with the problem, and more generally, to assess the individual's motivation and potential cooperation in various potential treatment plans. All of this should lead to a recommendation of an appropriate intervention plan to help the individual with his or her problem. These plans, depending on the nature of the assessment, can range from referring the patient to different agencies for specific help with such problems as financial support or legal aid to recommendations for various forms of supportive, individual, or group therapy. A complete assessment interview should always lead to a formulation of the nature of the problem and a recommendation that is realistic in terms of alleviating the difficulty and treating the individual. As was stated earlier, often the treatment process is and should be started even as the assessment process is taking place.

Actions taken and recommendations

The report should indicate what actions were taken during the assessment interview, for example, arranging for medication or finding a place for the person to stay. The interviewer's recommendations for the patient, including return appointments, should also be noted.

Evaluation Interview Report

Outline

I. *Identifying Information*

   1. *Name:* _____

   2. *Address and Phone No.:* _____

   _____

   3. *Date of Birth:* _____

   4. *Date and Place of Interview:* _____

   5. *Housing and Family Situation:* _____

   _____

    6. *Education:* _____

    7. *Occupation:* _____

    8. *Marital Status:* _____

    9. *No. of Children:* _____

   10. *Interviewer's Name:* _____

II. *Reason for Referral and Referral Source*
(Indicate clearly why the patient is being seen and who referred the patient to the service.)

III. *Patient's Statement and View of the Problem*
(Briefly explain how the patient sees the difficulty and what the patient thinks is wrong. Use patient's own words whenever possible.)

IV. *Information About the Problem from Other Sources*

(List other information about what is wrong that has come from other reports.)

V. *Behavior and Description of the Patient During Interview*

(Describe general appearance, dress, mood, feelings expressed, way client relates to interviewer, logic, emotional control, style of speech, etc.)

VI. *Precipitating Factors and the Patient's Immediate Situation*

(Describe the immediate life situation that set off the problem.)

VII. *Social and Developmental History* (When needed)

(Describe family background, early development, school, relationships, previous problems and difficulties. Include cultural and tribal factors that may be of importance.)

VIII. *Medical History* (When needed)

(Describe current and previous illness, medication, general health, nutrition, etc.)

IX. *Assessment Formulation of the Problem*

(Give your impressions about what is wrong and note the factors contributing to the problem.)

X. *Actions Taken and Recommendations*

(Indicate what steps were taken to deal with the problem and give recommendations for further help.)

Case records and reports

Maintaining a confidential record of the information about the patient is usually an important part of good handling of cases. It is often useful for the interviewer to summarize the main points of the case in a written report. Just by organizing all the information on the patient the interviewer can often better understand the patterns and implications of the information. In addition, having this information available in the case record will save much time and effort when the patient is seen by someone else at the clinic or returned after a long absence. There are many situations in which a knowledge of the patient's emotional difficulties will be very helpful when the patient is treated for a medical problem.

Two examples of brief assessment reports follow. Case 1 was written by an indigenous behavioral health technician. The referral was from a school about a girl who was absent frequently. Case 2 was written by a more experienced mental health professional and was about a young woman who had been referred by the court for neglect of her child. In order to protect the confidential nature of the case material, changes have been made in certain details to disguise the patient's identity.

EVALUATION INTERVIEW REPORT

CASE 1

Identifying information

Name: Jane
Address:
Age: 8 years
Occupation: Student
Education: Primary student

Date: September 8, 1975
Children:
Home Situation: Living at home
with mother
Interviewed by: Paraprofessional
Mental Health Practitioner in
Training

Referral source and reason

Jane was referred to us by Miss X, advisor for the Minority Education Department. Miss X stated that Jane had been regularly absent from school at least once a week, sometimes three times a week. Because of this she was not coping with her schoolwork.

Patient's statement of the problem

Jane is eight years old. She stated that she likes school and only stays away when she is sick. Further, she said that her mother takes her to the hospital when she is this way. When she was asked what kind of sickness she had, Jane replied that she was always having nosebleeds. She does not like to stay home because she has no friends to play with. Her sister is grown up (this woman is actually her mother) and she said she has a brother and a baby sister too. Her father died but she does not remember him. She likes watching television, especially wrestling, and also likes to watch Sesame Street and cartoons. Jane said that there is a baby at home and that her mother looks after him.

Information from other sources

Mother's statement of the problem   Jane's mother stated that Jane has been a sick girl. She has had some kind of rash all over her body for a whole year. She took Jane to the doctor but the doctor never gave her any medicine. He just said it will go away by itself. So her mother used to use her own medicine on her. It was something like coconut oil and it made her better. Her mother said she has been sick since she has been here. Last week she had a nosebleed and stayed home. Mother states Jane only stays home when she is sick.

Principal's statement of the problem   Mr. Y, principal of the school, stated that since Jane has been absent from school her school grades have been going down. Her academic achievement tests showed that her spelling and reading were at a lower level than average. When she spoke she sometimes tried to use big words but didn't really know what they meant. In her reading Jane realized that she could not read as well as the other children in her group. At one time she remarked that she must come to school more often so that she could read as well as the rest of the group. Mr. Y remarked that Jane has a very good sense of humor. She also gets on very well with her fellow students.

Behavior and description of patient

Jane seemed relaxed while talking to me. Sometimes she fiddled with her hands, but she always answered each question. Although her teacher said that Jane had a very loud voice and that one would always know when she was around, she spoke to us very quietly and sometimes she seemed shy. Her thinking was clear although difficult at coming to the point at times. Jane was dressed in old, shabby clothes. She observed a checker game with other children. She did not seem to understand the game at all.

Social history

Jane's mother is really her grandmother, as she adopted her as a baby. Jane believes her real mother is her sister. She has actually a younger brother and sister. Jane was born in a rural area and was five when she came to her current home and started school here. Jane was very bright as a baby. She walked before she was one and talked early. She is very helpful around the house. She goes to bed about eight o'clock every night and nearly always wakes by herself. Her mother never really has to wake her. Her mother never really forces her to go to school; if she complains of being a little sick her mother lets her stay home. She has plenty of white friends at home to play with, but only plays with colored children at school. Jane's home is an old style house. The front door was broken. The house was very clean and there appeared to be no fancy furniture around.

Medical history

None available.

Formulation of the problem and recommendation

Jane's mother is not really strict about her going to school. If she complains of a slight ache or pain she just lets her stay home. As Jane really likes school, all she needs is a little push from her mother and she will probably attend school regularly. At the present her mother does not care if she goes or not. Her mother stated that if Jane gets sick regularly she will bring her into the Medical Center to see the doctor. We will follow up in her attendance and work with her mother if she continues to miss school.

EVALUATION INTERVIEW REPORT
CASE 2
Identifying information

Name: Lillian Y.
Address:
Telephone No.:
Age: 18
Date of Birth:
Occupation: Has never worked
Education: Ninth grade

Date:
Marital Status: Single
Children: One
Home Situation: Lives with grandmother in a home with several aunts and uncles. The house is very crowded and needs repair.
Interviewed by: Experienced Mental Health Practitioner

Referral source and reason

Lillian was referred to the mental health agency by the court. She was charged by her grandmother with whom she lives of neglecting her one-year-old daughter. The court requested that Lillian be evaluated with regard to her ability to care for the child.

Patient's statement of the problem

Lillian indicated that her home situation was a very difficult one because there was constant arguing and fighting. She said that she frequently has arguments, especially with one uncle. This so upsets her that she will leave home and stay with friends for several days. When she does this Lillian does not take her baby girl along, but assumes that she will be taken care of by someone in the house. Lillian did not show any real indication of strong concern about or feeling of responsibility for the child when she goes away. Lillian did indicate that she gets little pleasure from playing with her baby, but did insist that feeding and caring for her was something which she liked to do.

Behavior and description of patient

Lillian was neat and appropriately dressed in casual clothes. She was somewhat shy, but was responsive and seemed to want to answer questions as best as she could. Her answers were often very simple and given without much thought or detail, but she was logical and did not get off the subject.

Precipitating factors and patient's current situation

It would appear that Lillian's neglect of her child primarily results from her leaving the household when she feels she can no longer take the tension, fighting, and arguments among family members. A particularly angry relationship with her only slightly older uncle has recently developed and this appears to be the main factor which has led her to leave home much more often than was true a few months ago. Further, the baby is now walking and is much more difficult to care for than she was when she was younger. The grandmother feels that the baby is more than she can deal with right now. The grandmother is elderly and not in very good health.

Social history

Lillian is the third of seven children. Her parents separated when she was a little over two years of age, and she has never really known her father. There was a great deal of marital tension when she was smaller. Both parents drank and frequently their arguments would end with her father beating her mother. Lillian's mother moved in with her mother, the present grandmother, and left much of the care of Lillian to grandmother and the others. Her mother continued to drink, had a succession of boyfriends, and three additional children who were fostered out among other relatives. The mother was killed in an automobile accident when Lillian was fourteen.

Lillian was always a very shy, timid, almost frightened girl who attended school until the ninth grade but never did well. She was placed in special education programs from the fifth grade on. She dropped out of school when she was sixteen in the ninth grade, and she became pregnant soon thereafter from a boy she knew briefly. Lillian showed little interest in the pregnancy and the new baby. She more and more seemed to expect the grandmother to care for and raise the child. However, she does do the things for the infant that grandmother tells her to do.

Lillian has a few friends in the general neighborhood, but other than going to them when she leaves home, she has no other social contacts. She is basically very shy, inhibited, and seems to have few interests or skills. Lillian achieved very poorly in school, reads only the simplest words, and has poor understanding of what's going on outside her immediate family situation.

Medical history

Lillian was a normal birth but did not thrive well. When she was three months of age it was thought that she was malnourished, and there was some evidence that she might have been beaten when she was about a year and a half. Socially she seemed to develop very slowly and to be a very retiring, clinging, dependent child, but with no major health problems.

Preliminary formulation of the problem

Lillian appears to be a shy, withdrawn, emotionally immature, and dependent young woman. Her living situation is apparently fraught with much arguing and tension which Lillian is unable to deal with and responds by leaving the situation for days at a time. She apparently expects that her child will be cared for by her grandmother and does not seem at this time to feel a great deal of involvement or responsibility for the baby.

Lillian appears to function intellectually in a rather limited way, and her capacity for understanding complex situations and her ability to learn need to be assessed. Basically she seems to be having considerable difficulty in accepting the responsibilities in bringing up her baby.

Actions taken and recommendations

It is recommended that Lillian be given an opportunity for counseling with regard to her feelings about her child and her child's care. Perhaps some direction and instruction regarding child care would be useful. It's also recommended that a less conflicted, tension-laden living situation should be found for Lillian. Since Lillian at this point seems dependent and immature, she probably needs to be in a situation where there will be some steady guidance and supervision. She should be given the opportunity to develop some vocational skills and a chance to increasingly become more independent in order to be able to provide more care for herself and for her infant.

The basis of her limited intellectual functioning needs to be assessed and thorough psychological testing of her potential and her achievement levels is recommended. Perhaps she should be given the opportunity for vocational training. The level at which she would be capable still needs to be determined.

She is in need of support in a helpful relationship which counseling could bring her. At the present time Lillian doesn't seem ready to independently care for her child. Depending on the outcome of the further evaluation with counseling and other forms of training, she may be able to function more independently. It is recommended that that course be followed and only if it does not turn out to be effective should other arrangements be made for her child's care.

Therapy or intervention interview

There are a wide range of intervention methods and psychotherapies that are carried out primarily through interviews. It is not the purpose of this section to attempt to describe in detail how these various therapy methods proceed in their particular approach to interviewing and working with patients. But we will discuss some general forms of intervention approaches that use interviews and later we will take up a few therapy interview methods in more detail.

Supportive therapy interview

When the assessment of a case indicates that the patient is in need of and will benefit from a primarily supportive therapy, the type of interviewing involved in this approach is that of listening to and understanding the patient. The therapist communicates to the patient an understanding of the patient's feelings and situation. Supportive therapy may also involve providing the patient with reassurance about the patient's ability to survive the difficult circumstances he or she is experiencing and about the patient's capability for solving the problem and being able to develop effective actions or providing support for directions and actions the patient has already taken.

Often in supportive therapy the therapist makes suggestions and advises the patient about things the patient can do through the patient's own actions with other people or about where and how to obtain assistance from various other available community resources. For instance, the therapist might suggest that the patient talk with her child's teacher, or advise her to apply for food stamps.

Thus, the therapist uses supportive interviews to listen to the patient and understand how the patient feels and what the patient's situation is. The therapy interview provides a safe place for the patient to express innermost thoughts and feelings. The therapist in a supportive role provides reassurance and suggests new directions and resources for the patient. Encouraging and facilitating the expression of feeling when emotional discharge is indicated or helping the patient to suppress and control feelings when that is necessary are both important aspects of the supportive interview.

Directive interview

Another type of intervention interview is the instructional, advice-giving, directive interview. When the assessment indicates that this approach is indicated the interviewer has a very active role in providing information, advice, and direction to the patient. In order for such information to be effective, the conditions of the interview must make sure that the patient is relaxed enough, motivated enough, and generally ready to use the information that the interviewer provides. It is important that the interviewer develop the proper conditions for relating to the patient so that the patient can accept the information that is given.

Directive interviews involve situations such as those in which the primary immediate problem has to do with legal rights and options, as might be the case in a crisis marriage situation. Informing such a patient about his or her general rights and how to go about obtaining proper legal advice and counsel would be an example of the kind of information imparted in such an interview. Another example of the use of the directive interview would be a situation in which a teen-ager simply did not have correct information on human sexuality and reproduction. Much of the teen-ager's difficulty and anxiety could be resolved by receiving correct information.

Self-understanding approaches

The third general type of therapy interview aims to help the patient gain increased awareness and understanding of himself or herself and of his or her behavior. There are a wide variety of therapy methods whose goal is to produce self-understanding, but each method may go about it differently. These techniques involve helping a person to attend to his or her immediate feelings and sensations, sometimes by developing situations in therapy so that these feelings will be forced to come about. Such approaches often help an individual to feel understood and comfortable with his or her feelings and to be more realistic in a self-appraisal. Furthermore, self-understanding interviews may confront individuals with the implications of their feelings, verbalizations, and actions, or they may help them see the relationship between past experiences and conflicts and current feelings and behaviors. The purpose of the self-understanding interview is to allow the individual to put self-understanding into action so that he or she can improve his or her situation and be more effective. The emphasis in this interview is to help the patient to take responsibility and act in his or her own interest instead of depending on the instruction, direction, or support of the therapist.

In order to be effective with any of these intervention interviews, it is important for the therapist to understand the purpose and goals of the method he or she is using. It is especially important to have mastered the interviewing techniques of a particular method in order to use it effectively.

Standardized versus open-form interview

A standardized interview is an interview in which questions are determined and written down before the interview begins. During the interview each question is asked in the exact wording in which it was written and in the exact order in which the questions were listed. The standardized interview is convenient for the interviewer because it covers the areas needed and the wording of each question is such that the answer can be compared to the answers of others who have been asked the same question in the same way. The standardized interveiw is most usually used in situations in which the purpose of the interview is to obtain research data. Sometimes it is used by interviewers who have not yet learned the skills of their task.

For clinical purposes, the standardized interview is generally not very useful. In most cases, interviewers have already determined the purpose or goal for the interview and have in mind some general areas and questions they want to cover. Rarely, if ever, would they do so in such a rigidly standard manner. The reason that an open-form interview is usually used in a clinical situation is because it establishes rapport and empathy with the patient. Open-form interviews allow patients to express themselves fully in their own terms and in the way that they conceptualize their problems and not in the way that standard questions might force answers. Nevertheless, the interviewer should be aware of standardized interviews and the fact that for some purposes they can be useful.

Confidentiality and privileged communication

Trust is one of the fundamental elements of effective clinical interviewing and any clinical work. Patients, after all, are suffering from severe and painful feelings or situations which almost always are very personal and ordinarily are considered private. Concerns and feelings about confidentiality must be dealt with in order for effective evaluations and therapy to take place. Unless the patient can feel certain that what he or she tells the interviewer will be kept private and confidential and only be used in helping him or her with the difficulty, the patient ordinarily will not reveal himself or herself. Consequently, adequate assessment and effective treatment may be hindered.

For these reasons, information and conclusions about the patient must be kept confidential in the same way that medical records are ordinarily kept confidential in a physician's or a hospital's records.

The nature of any limits to confidentiality that may be the case in any particular setting that a patient comes to should be made clear to the patient before he or she starts to reveal himself or herself. When most people come to see a doctor or come to a health clinic they can assume fairly that information about them and about their conditions will be kept confidential. However, there are cases in which this may not be so, and the patient should be informed of that before agreeing to give information.

First, it must be recognized that when a patient is being seen in a clinic the confidentiality usually means that the information is confidential within the clinic and not confidential just between the patient and the interviewer. For instance, in most clinic operations the interviewer staffs the case, which means that those members of the clinic who are concerned will hear about the case and participate in the recommendations for the case. Also, the interviewer's or therapist's supervisor may want to hear about the case. Persons in clinics and hospitals who have no professional involvement in the case would not ordinarily be informed about the case.

Utmost caution must be taken in discussing cases and in the care of case records. Cases should only be discussed with those persons who have a legitimate reason for knowing about the case and only under conditions in which information about the case will not be overheard or carelessly revealed. Generally, cases should only be discussed during professional meetings. They should never be discussed at family or social gatherings.

Limits to confidentiality

There are some cases in clinical work in which information about the patient is not confidential. When the patient cannot be guaranteed confidentiality for what he or she tells the interviewer, the interviewer should make clear before starting the interview what the conditions and limitations of confidentiality are.

Confidentiality does not hold when the patient is referred for an evaluation by an agency that requests a detailed report on the patient's condition. For example, the court may want to know about a person's condition for trial purposes or for considering placement or other measures. Schools sometimes request evaluations of children, with the understanding that the reports will be sent back to the school. Under these circumstances, the interviewer's good judgment determines what is important and useful for the report on an interview evaluation. For example, the interviewer may decide to leave out some sensitive things that have no real bearing on the questions asked for the evaluation. Nonetheless, the interviewer may not legally be able to maintain confidentiality if he or she were pressed on the matter, since confidentiality was not a condition of that particular interview.

Confidentiality is not maintained when the patient may be a danger to himself or herself or to others. Thus, if the confidential information indicates that there is a reasonable likelihood of the patient's doing serious harm to himself or herself or to someone else, such information is not kept confidential. Rather, the information must be used for the protection of the person or for the protection of society. Ordinarily, this information should be reported only after it is thoroughly discussed with the patient and the patient is told why the information is being reported. However, these are usually emergency situations and it is not always possible or practical to handle it this way.

Privileged communication

Information given in confidence by a patient is called privileged communication. In most countries, certain groups are permitted by law or custom to withhold information told them in confidence, even from courts of laws. In Western countries these are often attorneys with regard to their clients' communications, religious leaders with regard to parishioners, and physicians with regard to patients. The privilege means, however, that it is up to the patient to decide whether or not information about him or her can be released. It is not the privilege of the one who has gathered the information. Rather, it is the patient who has the right to decide whether or not information about himself or herself may be released by the doctor, lawyer, or other person who has access to it.

Frequently, the patient who has been seen at a clinic or office may at sometime in the future require evaluation or treatment at another clinic or office. It is, of course, very useful in making a new evaluation to know what a person's condition was in the past. The new agency will ordinarily wish to request the information about the person that is available from the earlier contact. In order for the first agency to release this information, permission must be obtained from the patient. This is usually done at the patient's request and the patient signs a release to the new agency. If there is no release, however, the patient's confidential records may not be released because the privilege of this communication is the patient's and not the agency's.

Styles and approaches

There is no single or exact way to approach a clinical interview. Interviewers, after all, are individual people with their own styles of doing things based on the ways they have learned to communicate and interact with others, based on the particular ways they have of viewing people and understanding them, and based on how they see the purpose of the interviews. This is not to say, however, that interviewers do not follow general guidelines. Rather, this is meant to convey that even within these guidelines there is room for interviewers to develop ways of interviewing with which they are most comfortable and which seem most natural.

As we shall see, being genuine is one important factor in developing therapy relationships. To try to relate in ways in which the interviewer is uncomfortable or ways that seem unnatural to the interviewer may indeed make for less than satisfactory clinical interviews.

The other crucially important factor that determines the style and approach of the interview lies in the patient who is being interviewed. The interview is, after all, an interactive process even if one person takes the responsibility for maintaining the direction toward its purpose. The interviewer's style must remain flexible and responsive to the patient whether the patient is very angry and resistant to the purposes of the interview, or the patient is severely depressed and unresponsive, or the patient is very suspicious. This again is a very important reason why a set formula, routine way of interviewing cannot be precisely set forth and probably should not be used even if such a way of doing it could be worked out.

Some basic elements of clinical interviewing

Obviously, the usefulness of the clinical interview depends very crucially on the participation, cooperation, and involvement of the patient. A successful interview must involve the patient in a meaningful way and it must provide an atmosphere in which the patient can feel free to express himself or herself openly. There are a number of factors that bring about a successful clinical interview. Most of these have to do with the interpersonal relationship developed between the interviewer and the patient, but some of them are also a function of the purpose and situation in which both parties find themselves in the interview. One such factor is the professional status the patient attributes to the interviewer. Another is the patient's confidence in how the material he or she exposes will be dealt with and handled by the interviewer. The issue of confidentiality is an important aspect here.

Developing the kind of relationship between the patient and the therapist that will facilitate a successful interview requires both skill and effort on the part of the interviewer. That quality of relationship is often described in terms of the *rapport* between the people or the *empathy* that exists between them. Both terms convey the idea of a situation in which both parties, but especially the patient because the patient is the main focus, feel comfortable, accepted, and in emotional touch with each other. It is very satisfying to feel understood by someone with whom one is willing and wants to share his or her feelings.

Factors that enhance and encourage the development of interview rapport and empathy have in many respects already been identified. One such important factor is that the interviewer treat the patient with *respect and dignity*. This involves the interviewer's accepting the person as a basically worthwhile human being regardless of the person's current status in life, the person's current problems or maladaptive responses, and regardless of what the person might have done. First, this does not mean that the interviewer approves of everything about the patient, but that the interviewer basically grants the patient the respect and dignity due a person who is struggling to deal with problems if only poorly or even antisocially. Second, the interviewer must convey his or her interests and willingness to understand the patient, including his or her feelings, and how he or she views the situation. The interviewer must communicate this understanding to the patient in such ways that the patient knows that he or she is being heard. Third, the interviewer must avoid taking a moralizing or punishing approach to the patient and the patient's problems. Instead, the interviewer must accept the patient's behavior as part of the patient's situation and must work to understand it. Fourth, the interviewer must maintain a professional role during the interview by providing and ensuring confidentiality when that is indicated, by maintaining a focus and goal for the interview, by focusing on the problems of the patient and not bringing up his or her own problems, and by carrying out the role of one who is knowledgeable and trained so that he or she will be perceived as a person from whom the patient can rightly expect help to reduce the suffering and help to solve his or her problems.

These then are factors which hopefully promote the patient's feelings of confidence and trust in the interviewer as a person who is understanding, is there to help and not criticize, who respects the patient despite whatever the patient's problems and weaknesses might be, who will maintain the confidentiality of the communication, and who is skilled and knowledgeable about what these things mean and how to deal with them.

To feel understood, respected by someone who is interested and has the skills to help, is indeed a powerful factor for developing effective rapport in clinical situations.

Genuineness, empathy, and warmth

Successful therapists who work with methods that primarily stress the relationship between the patient and the therapist are genuine, empathetic, and warm. *Genuineness* refers to sincerity. It is not merely playing a role or following a mechanical technique or pretending to be interested, understanding, and wanting to be of help to the patient. Rather, it means being open and real, being interested, having respect for the patient, and really wanting to help.

Successful therapists have the ability to communicate *accurate empathy*. That is, they have the ability to understand accurately the meanings and feelings of the patient and to communicate this understanding of the patient to the patient so that the patient can feel that what he or she says and how he or she feels is indeed getting through to a person who is interested.

The therapist conveys *nonpossessive warmth*, the feeling of liking and acceptance of the person with whom he or she is working. This liking is, however, not dependent on the person's doing only what the therapist wants, and it is not a jealous possessiveness or used as a way to direct or force the person to do what the therapist wants. Rather, it is a notion of liking because the other individual is a human being worthy of being liked and respected.

Genuineness, empathy, and warmth are of particular importance in therapy interviews, but they are also important in any clinical interview. Interviewers should strive to increasingly develop them in order to form more effective relationships with those with whom they work.

Interviewers should keep in mind that a clinical interview always has a purpose and a more or less specifiable goal. In general, the purpose of the interview is to assess the individual and the individual's situation, for treatment, or for follow-up. While the interviewer should not be entirely rigid with regard to what he or she sees is the goal of the interview, it is important that focus is maintained so that the interview generally will proceed in a productive direction toward some clear means of helping the patient.

Some useful techniques for interviewing

The interviewer, of course, talks to the patient. The interviewer makes statements, asks questions, and responds to the patient's communications. For the interviewer, the interview is not an offhand procedure but a procedure based on an overall goal and direction. It is that goal and direction that keep the interview from becoming a confused, purposeless series of mixed contradictory communications. But having a goal and direction is not enough for a good clinical interview. There must also be some particular technique or means by which the interviewer can reach the goal, direction, and purpose of the interview. Below are described some interview techniques that may be useful in a variety of situations. Their usefulness depends on the goal of the interview.

Conveying interest and understanding

A generally useful overall technique in interviewing, one that will be particularly useful in developing rapport and empathy, a basic necessity for most interviewing, is that of conveying to the patient that the interviewer is interested in the patient as a person. This can be done by paying respectful attention to the patient and what the patient has to say, and particularly by sensitively trying to understand what the patient is feeling and what it must be like for the patient. From time to time the interviewer needs to communicate to the patient what the interviewer understands of what the patient has expressed. In this way, the interviewer clearly indicates that he or she is trying to understand

and can check the accuracy of his or her understanding. If the interviewer's understanding is not right, this then gives the patient the chance to clear it up. Then accurate communication can continue. The interviewer can develop an understanding of the patient's experience by asking such appropriately timed questions as, "How did that make you feel?" or "That must have made you very angry." It is also useful for the interviewer to let the patient know when he or she is unsure about the meaning of what the patient has said. This can be done by statements such as, "I'm not sure I really understand about that," or "How do you feel about it?" or "Tell me more about that situation."

When people feel that there is someone who is interested and wants to understand what it is like for them, they usually feel much freer to express their feelings more openly and more readily than they would otherwise. Thus, both the attitude and responses which show interest and the desire to understand the person demonstrate that the interviewer is listening to the patient, considers what the patient is saying is important, and also is accepting it without criticism. The interviewer can do this by saying things to let the patient know that he or she has listened and tried to understand. By occasionally summarizing what he or she understands, the interviewer can make sure that he or she correctly understands what the patient means.

It is often useful to ask open-ended and nonjudgmental questions such as, "Tell me about your father," "What do you plan to do?" and "Tell me more about that." These may open up important areas of needed information without putting the patient on the defensive or on guard.

Usually, a useful approach is to follow the patient's lead and develop questions from what the patient has indicated is his or her concern. But this needs to be done without losing the direction, purpose, and goal of the interview. Therefore, when important areas have not been brought up by the patient, the interviewer may have to bring them up by saying just enough to help the patient to begin to bring up the needed information. The interviewer should not shift the heavy responsibility for the verbalization in the interview from the patient. Rather, the interviewer should encourage the patient to express things fully in his or her own way and on his or her own terms. The context in which this should be done is a setting in which rapport and empathy are well established.

Nonverbal communication and body language

When interviewing one should be aware that a great deal of communication goes on between people in addition to whatever words are spoken (Birdwhistell, 1970). In fact, it well may happen that the behavior or voice tone or the way in which something is said communicates an entirely different message from what the words have said. The popular term for this nonverbal communication is body language. There are many individual ways of expressing things in body language. The interviewer should carefully observe the patient's actions; for example, how the patient sits, stands, and moves and whether or not the patient looks at the interviewer. Such things as crossing the legs or arms, tapping the fingers, or stroking the hair can be important, especially when they seem to occur more frequently when certain feelings or topics come up. Leaning forward and looking at someone suggests that one is interested in the person. Pulling back or looking away suggests disinterest. There can be slumped, dejected positions and angry, defiant positions.

There is an interesting study on how adolescent girls behaved in an interview led by a man and depending on whether or not they had lost their fathers. When the father's absence was due to death, the girls often seemed frightened of men. But when the father's absence was due to divorce, the girls were more likely to act seductively toward the male interviewer.

Being aware of these body language clues in the interview makes for a much more effective interviewer and an interview that can more effectively do what it is intended to do.

summary

1 The interview is the basic tool of mental health work. It requires special social communication skills and is not the same as social communication.

2 The clinical interviewer has a definite goal, that of helping the patient. The interviewer must direct the interview toward the goal, facilitate communication, focus on the patient's problems, and make the arrangements.

3 Clinical interviews are of several types: The assessment interview focuses on understanding the problems, strengths, and weaknesses of the patient and formulating recommendations. The therapy interview can be supportive and involves listening, understanding, reassuring, and giving directions and suggestions. The directive interview involves mostly instruction, advice, or directions in situations in which the person isn't capable of functioning without it. The self-understanding interview works to help the patient achieve increased self-awareness.

4 Trust is essential to clinical interviewing, and confidentiality is crucial. There are some circumstances, due either to the nature of the referral or to the life-threatening situation, in which confidentiality does not apply.

5 Some basic factors in successful clinical interviewing center on establishing a warm, trusting communication. This is enhanced by showing the patient respect and dignity, by being genuine, empathetic, and warm, and by conveying interest and understanding.

6 Communication is not only verbal; it is also nonverbal. Understanding body language is an important aspect of the interviewer's skill.

Crisis treatment and suicide prevention: Intervention and therapy

Crisis intervention and/or therapy are usually the best means for dealing with severe situational emotional problems. Things move to a peak in a crisis, and a turning point for better or for worse is inevitable. Therefore, quick and accurate action is important. A main goal of crisis work is to defuse the crisis by assisting the patient to take actión toward the most favorable alternative outcome available and to prevent actions or inactions that could lead to negative consequences.

The crisis situation is different in several ways from other forms of mental health problems. Crisis is characterized by the immediate urgency of the situation, the emergency nature of the intervention procedures that need to be carried out. These procedures are performed in the context of a limited contact because of the brief period of time available in which to take effective action. A crisis situation is distinguished from other situations in which the immediate problem is less urgent and unstable, or in which concern about a disastrous outcome is not as immediate, or in which there is enough time to use more thorough and less emergency methods.

In some ways, however, both crisis intervention and crisis therapy are types of short-term therapy. Many of the techniques and approaches used in crisis work originated and have been borrowed from other sources. Rather than being any single, well-defined method, crisis therapy and intervention are better thought of as special ways of looking at emergency problems and their alleviation. Many different methods are brought in to deal with crisis situations.

Approaching crisis

Crisis treatment should not be viewed simply as an expedient patchup or a finger-in-the-dyke type of first aid treatment, although sometimes it can be just that. Rather, the theory of crisis intervention considers the successful coming through and mastering of a crisis as something that can have a very positive result. This can happen if, through successfully handling the crisis, the individual learns new and more effective ways of coping and dealing with future problem situations. Some even go so far as to say that it is only through experiencing and successfully resolving crises that people learn how to move to a positive and effective adjustment.

Types of crisis

Crises can and do occur for everyone at some periods in their lifetime. *Developmental crises* are crises experienced by all people as they progress through the various life stages. Developmental crises occur at change points in life. At such times people must master new situations and circumstances and learn new means of coping with both the outside world and their own internal feelings and capabilities. Many people, probably most, come through their development crises without unusual stress and strain. They make effective choices that will be adaptive and move them ahead in their developmental cycle. But for others, the developmental crises are times of great difficulty and cause extreme stress with which they are unable to adequately cope and deal. Poor solutions to developmental crises can lead to greater stress, and they may result in severe deterioration of effectiveness and control of emotions and behavior.

Some of the more crucial developmental crisis points, which may or may not turn out to be special problems for individuals, start as early as weaning from the breast or the bottle to solid foods. For some infants, this is a serious adjustment crisis. Toilet training is frequently a problem for many children and their parents. Adolescence, of course, is a period of great stress and need for adjustment. Pubescent persons must cope with great changes in their bodies and impulses and in the demands made on them by their culture and society. Similarly, the stages of menopause and aging often are stressful and call for adjustments and choice of positive alternatives and actions so as to avoid the negative results of these conditions. For many people, these changes and the adjustments needed are not terribly intense and they happen slowly over time. But for others, they build as crises to intense, desperate, and anxious conflicts that must be resolved without delay.

Accidental crises are situations and events which happen to people, sometimes with little or no involvement on their part. For example, the sudden death of a mother, father, child, or spouse may precipitate an intense crisis associated with the grief and the loss. Similarly, other kinds of losses may result in crisis reactions. These include loss of a job, failure in school, the breakup of a marriage or a love affair, natural disasters (for example, fire destroying one's home, flood, storms which take away all the possessions an individual might have), or an illness or accident which may suddenly change an individual's way of life (e.g., a soccer player who is injured and can no longer walk, or a seamstress whose eyesight fails and who can no longer sew).

Crises, however, cannot be defined only in terms of what has happened or changed in an individual's life. Rather, the crisis must be defined by the individual when the individual feels overwhelmed and unable to successfully deal with the situation by the means the individual has used for past problems and when the individual is not at that point able to develop new effective means of coping with the situation.

When crisis treatment is indicated

People in crisis experience great anxiety, confusion, desperation, fear, helplessness, and hopelessness. Intervention measures must quickly and accurately assess the situation and decisively deal with it. Crises don't wait until full detailed histories are taken, or until one's turn comes up on the treatment waiting list, or until an ideal therapy relationship develops with the therapist.

Rather, people in crisis states are in desperate need. Usually, they feel in desperate need and are seeking help for right now and are at that point open to receive help. For some, this may be the only time when they are responsive to intervention. In this case, crisis intervention can sometimes be the best means to effectively and positively influence the individual's future adjustment. It may be realistically the only point at which the individual can be helped to make changes and adjustments in his or her life and behavior.

Effectiveness with lower socioeconomic persons

It is well known that many individuals of the lower socioeconomic strata do not respond well to most of the standard types of psychotherapy. The reasons for this are not entirely clear, but it seems that many lower socioeconomic people are much more amenable to help when in crisis situations and do benefit at such times from a crisis approach. One of the observed factors in this is that many lower socio-economic individuals are not likely to seek help until the situation is of crisis proportions. Furthermore, the help they seek is direct relief. Once the acute stress has been alleviated, they generally are unlikely to return for further work on the less crucially immediate aspects of their problems. This pattern is certainly not true of all lower socioeconomic people, but is for many. Crisis intervention has thus been viewed as an especially well-suited method for dealing with lower socioeconomic individuals because it provides them with help and assistance during their periods of intense difficulty.

Development of the crisis method

Crisis treatment, as an important treatment method in its own right, is fairly recent. In World War II it was found that brief treatment for soldiers who were under the extreme stress of war was effective because it allowed the individual to stay with his unit, preserve his self-esteem, and avoid the sense of guilt about leaving his buddies. Thus, crisis treatment was found not only effective for the crisis but also useful as a preventive. This approach was next used for dealing with acute grief reactions as, for example, when there was the sudden loss of a loved one.

Lindemann (1944), who developed much of the early technique of crisis work, has described some of the patterns typical of crisis. First, there is usually an acute onset with a clear situation that sets it off. Second, since the choices of action that can be taken, either positive or negative, are usually few, the outcome of each action is often predictable. Third, the symptoms of crisis stress usually are temporary and not the sign of a major lasting mental disorder. Fourth, the steps necessary to deal emotionally with each situation feeding the crisis can be specified.

Much of Lindemann's work has been influential in the further development of crisis therapy. Suicide prevention and the development of suicide prevention and crisis centers are outgrowths of his work.

Stages of crisis reaction

According to Caplan (1964), a crisis is experienced by an individual as an intense upset, which results from that individual's inability to deal with the situation by the coping methods that have worked successfully for the individual in the past. The immediate crisis reaction is followed by a time of disorganization and confusion, and, generally, attempts to deal with the problem are ineffective. Within four to six weeks, according to Caplan, an outcome, either positive or negative, occurs.

The four phases of a crisis are as follows: (1) When the crisis develops, the individual experiences tension and disorganization and tries to manage the situation using his or her previous ways of dealing with problems. (2) If that fails, more disorganization, anxiety, and confusion occur. (3) Tension increases greatly and the individual seeks to bring to bear internal and external resources. This includes seeking help at this point or changing his or her goal. (4) If these efforts fail to resolve the crisis, then the person may become extensively disorganized and emotional breakdown may occur.

Levels of intervention

Interventions in crisis situations may be considered at four different levels. The first level is termed *environmental manipulation* in which the role of the crisis intervener is really that of a referral source to put the individual in touch with the appropriate resources. For example, if the crisis focus is around a family that has been evicted from their home and have no place to stay or have no money for food, the crisis intervener makes sure that the troubled person gets to the appropriate sources for help.

The second level of crisis intervention is called *general support.* This involves the crisis therapist's listening and providing an accepting, nonthreatening, encouraging relationship and a safe outlet for feeling. For example, if an individual has suddenly lost a loved one, the therapist's approach would be to listen sympathetically and respectfully and give encouragement about the future.

The third level of crisis intervention, *combined approach,* is one in which the helper can bring to bear both general knowledge of crisis situations as well as of specific kinds of methods and approaches that are effective for resolving them. For instance, a family crisis precipitated by a pregnancy and an unmarried early teen-age daughter may be dealt with by support and eliciting emotional catharsis on the part of those concerned, by helping the family members to face the reality of the situation and then exploring the alternatives, and then finally by helping them to make a decision.

A fourth level of crisis intervention involves a strategy which in addition to the other methods includes developing some *deeper understanding of the personality of the individual.* These methods would include developing knowledge of the individual's personality, defensive styles, strengths and weaknesses, as well as broader aspects of the individual as a person. For instance, in the case of acute depression occurring after the loss of a loved one, the therapist would use knowledge of the patient's previous history of such losses and reactions to them. The previous patterns of coping with such situations may indicate what to expect in the present situation.

Crisis intervention and crisis therapy

Crises can be categorized into two general types. There are those which can be best handled by direction and direct actions, largely through some kind of environmental manipulation. This way of handling situations is what accurately might be called *crisis intervention*. If the situation is such that either the environmental manipulation by itself will handle the situation or if the individual is so incapacitated and ineffectual that he or she is not able to respond to crisis therapy, then environmental manipulation is the treatment of choice.

Crisis therapy, in contrast, involves helping the individual to resolve his or her own realistic choices and to effect a realistic solution to the situation. Crisis therapy, as has been noted, is a form of brief therapy. Typically, it runs from one to four or five sessions. Crisis therapy, as compared to crisis intervention, is used when the best resolution of the crisis calls for a decision by the patient and when the patient has some capability to act effectively in his or her situation by remobilizing coping mechanisms.

Crisis therapy rather than intervention should be used when most of the following aspects of the situation are present: (1) when the problem is resolvable and lies largely within the person, and within the capabilities of that individual to solve, rather than being a situation that can be handled with temporary aid from the outside; (2) when the person in crisis has the capability to explore the problem with the therapist in terms of the person's own responsibility for the situation; (3) when the individual is motivated to change things and has the ability to act on his or her own behalf; (4) when the individual is available to come in for treatment; (5) when the individual's personality makeup is such that a therapy relationship would be helpful rather than harmful (past history of previous treatment would be important in determining this factor); and (6) when the relative cost to benefit ratio is favorable, that is, would the benefit resulting from the investment of staff time in this individual situation be worth the expense? (Cost is a reality that must be considered, but humane case handling must always remain the primary consideration.)

Doing crisis work

The realistic goal of crisis work is to return the patient to a level of adjustment that the patient had before experiencing the crisis. Thus, the focus is very much on the here and now and dealing with the situation that precipitated the crisis. In crisis work there is little time for casual social chatter. Time must be used efficiently for dealing directly and firmly with what is going on.

The effective crisis therapist must have many skills and must be flexible. Almost simultaneously the therapist must diagnose the nature and extent of the problem, provide support, learn the facts, and develop interventions for dealing with the problem. Within a very short time in the first and very likely the only interview, the crisis therapist must accomplish a variety of things. The therapist must (1) develop a working relationship with the patient; (2) develop enough of the right information in order to work out a treatment plan; (3) consider the situation in terms of both the precipitating factors and the personality structure of the patient; (4) share with the patient a view of the problem that will include information that will help the patient to see both the maladaptive things that he or she is doing as well as those behaviors that are appropriate and effective; (5) help the patient to explore new and better or alternative ways of approaching the problem; (6) help the patient to find a new approach for achieving the goals that have been mutually agreed upon; and finally (7) arrange for any future interviews or recommend other agencies and resources that might be of use.

Qualifications of the crisis intervener

The qualifications needed for an individual to be an effective, helpful crisis intervener and therapist are essentially the same as for those who do sensitive and effective interviewing or other clinical work. The following have been stated as the basic abilities needed by successful interveners: (1) empathetic ability, that is, the capacity of the crisis therapist for understanding the problems that have been experienced by the patient; (2) the ability to listen carefully and selectively and to develop the necessary information from the patient who can't easily express himself or herself; (3) the ability to listen objectively and to avoid putting personal values and personal needs into the assessment or treatment; (4) the ability to assess and formulate the person's situation quickly and accurately; and (5) the ability to use the resources of the community to make the necessary referrals. In addition, sometimes some of these abilities are enhanced if the crisis intervener is a member of the same subculture as that of the troubled individual.

Since crisis therapy is very time limited and must deal with a whole range of things, from assessment through definitive decisions, in a very short period of time, the therapist must be very confident and skilled and usually must be very firm and direct in approach. The therapist should provide the patient with an image of someone who can understand the patient's problem and is human and concerned about the patient. At the same time, the crisis therapist must be very direct and focused in order to get to the information that is needed so quickly. Thus, in contrast to most other kinds of therapists, the crisis therapist must be very active and direct in the situation. The therapist must always be in command and able to size up the problem rapidly. The crisis therapist must be prepared, depending on the situation, to be supportive or confronting, to take over responsibility or to insist that the patient do so. Further, the crisis therapist must deal realistically with the patient and the patient's situation, often by giving specific feedback to the patient.

The therapist often needs to take firm, strong stands about situations and actions, both when supporting the patient's efforts or confronting the patient about unrealistic behaviors or when exploring realistic possibilities. The crisis therapist may have to set the goals and help the patient to find new ways and new approaches to consider.

Assessment of crisis

The basic information necessary for the assessment of crisis includes the same data and observations that are needed and gone into much more extensively in the more usual assessment interview. Some basic factual and background information, such as name, age, marital status, occupation, and so forth, is necessary. Much can be learned from observation of the patient's general appearance, how the patient is dressed, and how the patient behaves during the interview, as well as from the structure of the patient's speech and manner of expression, from the content of the patient's verbalizations, and from the patient's mood and emotional state. How the patient relates and responds to the interviewer is very informative. In addition, finding out about the patient's precrisis adjustment and how the patient has dealt with crises in the past can be very important. The emphasis, of course, should be on the current life pressures, but when they can be clearly tied to past problems, developing this information on them can be very useful.

One of the first things the crisis therapist must decide is whether or not the patient really can be adequately evaluated and whether or not a resolution can be found for the current state. If, for instance, the patient is overdosed on drugs or alcohol, or even if the individual is too agitated or physically exhausted to provide the necessary information, then the physical factors must be dealt with first. Obviously, in order for a minimally adequate evaluation of the problem to be made, a person has to be sufficiently calm and has to make enough sense to be able to provide the necessary information. When a person is too disturbed to be adequately evaluated, friends, family, or police may be able to provide information. A person in crisis may have to be watched or hospitalized until he or she becomes sufficiently cooperative and logical to evaluate.

Determining the patient's motivation for taking responsibility for his or her problems is necessary. The situation is different when the therapist is dealing with someone who is looking for magical help, perhaps feeling completely discouraged and helpless, and asking for miracles than when dealing with someone who is very dependent on the therapist but capable of cooperating and participating with the therapist. When the crisis therapist is working with an individual who wants help to figure out how to deal with the problem himself or herself, then the therapist can use a different approach and probably will have a much easier time of it. This patient should respond well to procedures that will work toward beneficial effects beyond the crisis problem.

Goals of crisis therapy and intervention

The primary goal of crisis treatment is to relieve the pressure on the individual and resolve the individual's immediate situation rather than aiming for more long-term or basic changes in personality or ways of dealing with things. In addition to relieving the presenting complaint or symptom, the crisis therapist first aims to steady the individual so that there will be no further disorganization and then to help the individual return to the level of adjustment that existed before the crisis. Most ideally, the aim would include helping the patient develop a more optimal level of functioning.

There are always stresses in the patient's life situation that can set off a crisis. When the crisis occurs, it is usually the last straw in a series of stresses. Understanding the stress that set off the crisis can help the therapist focus the intervention and therapy on this stress. Also, understanding the factors of the crisis from the individual's past history is often important in a successful resolution of the problem. It is also very helpful for the patient to understand his or her present reaction to the precipitating stress in light of some of the patient's past development and past ways of dealing with stresses.

Very often the only contact a therapist has with an individual in crisis is the one time that the individual is seen during the crisis situation. This is probably especially true when dealing with lower socioeconomic minority groups. In this case, the crisis interview should be conducted as if it will be the one and only available opportunity to work with the patient. A therapist, thus, has to rapidly evaluate the situation and make clear, decisive, and durable decisions that will lead to necessary actions.

Methods of crisis therapy

In crisis therapy, unlike in many other therapies, the therapist must play a very authoritative and direct role. The crisis therapist must be seen as an expert who has the power to help and give relief. In general, the therapist has a variety of methods for working with the crisis. These include attentive and understanding listening to the problem, providing reassurance and support for some behaviors, criticizing and redirecting other behaviors, giving advice, and bringing in outside agencies or dealing with relatives.

The crisis therapist provides emotional support and reassurance to the patient by communicating nonpossessive warmth and acceptance of the individual and by presenting a trustworthy, strong image on which the patient feels that he or she can rely.

The therapist also provides an opportunity for the patient to express and discharge feelings without fear of embarrassment or undue criticism. Being able to let out feelings, that is, to have an emotional catharsis, be it fear, rage, or other feelings, has long been recognized as an important technique in helping people who are emotionally upset.

The therapist needs to communicate an optimistic and hopeful outlook for the patient. Encouraging the patient that he or she has done the right thing by coming in for help, and that a workable solution for the situation is indeed possible, is a useful way of conveying hope.

The therapist needs to become very active and involved in the patient's problem situation. In addition, the therapist must attentively stay in touch with the patient's communication and with what is going on emotionally within the patient.

The therapist must develop skill in listening very selectively to the material the patient brings out and in keeping the focus of the interview on the basic crisis situation. It is important not to become diverted to side issues or situations which are not of close relevance to the crisis problem.

The therapist may often have to provide the patient with factual information about the problem and situation. This may have to do with misconceptions about things as diverse as sexuality, the hereditary nature of mental illness, or how to find out about and gain one's legal rights.

When sufficient information has been developed, then the crisis therapist, together with the patient, decides what the major problem situation is. They develop some possible goals and consider what means there are for achieving them. It is important that the patient be fully involved with this process and that, as much as possible, defining the problem, setting goals, and developing options be done jointly.

Some general things that the therapist should always keep in mind are to try to always be clear, definitive, and to the point in communications with the patient. The therapist should not hesitate to point out what some of the negative consequences could be if the patient does not take action, as well as what can be gained by making the necessary moves.

Giving advice and making direct suggestions are positive strategies when there is a good chance that the patient will take the advice and when there is a good possibility of success if the advised actions are taken. But if the patient resists taking advice, or if there is too much advice, or if the advice has little chance of working, the patient will lose confidence in the therapist.

In some circumstances, it is necessary for the therapist to set very clear limits on the patient's behavior. These limits may have to be very strict in situations of extreme danger to the patient or others. For example, the therapist should not hesitate to take firm action when a very disorganized borderline patient threatens to harm himself or herself or others.

The therapist should support those behaviors and actions that are adaptive and that are working or have worked in the past and should seek new alternative behaviors for those that aren't working. When the patient is unrealistic or has not come to grips with the reality of the situation, then confronting the patient directly and firmly with his or her unrealistic ideas or behavior is required.

The crisis therapist should devise a very definite plan and make specific suggestions for the patient. The therapist should also propose some very concrete requirements for the patient and should have the patient agree to carry them out. A therapeutic contract is often useful in this case. The contract can cover a range of issues, e.g., an agreement about further treatment or specific actions the patient agrees to carry out. The therapist should always be prepared to directly take action in the patient's situation. This might include enlisting the aid of friends, relatives, and employers.

In general, then, crisis intervention and crisis therapy are the first and foremost means of treatment of individuals who are experiencing acute difficulties. In another sense, however, the crisis intervention approach is as much a frame of reference for looking at mental health as a way to treat emotional difficulties. From that standpoint intervening at the time of crisis is a preventive tool as well as a treatment. It is preventive because it deals with the problem before it becomes chronic or before deterioration occurs. Success at resolving a crisis moves the patient on to positive personality development.

Many of the techniques used in crisis intervention and therapy are borrowed from other approaches. Rapid assessment, accurate diagnostic evaluation, and very direct active intervention based on the assessment are crucial in this method.

There are also many practical advantages to a crisis approach to treatment. Since there is a brief contact and there are few sessions, a small staff can see many more cases than can a clinic that uses more detailed evaluations and longer term treatment. Furthermore, the method seems effective and suitable for lower socioeconomic individuals and can be carried out successfully by paraprofessionals. Since indigenous workers of the lower socioeconomic community often are more effective than others, their use of the crisis approach appears to be the most suitable approach for the majority of cases of that group.

As has been noted, the nature of a crisis is always personal. In the end it must be defined by the individual who is experiencing the situation as stressful. Crises can also be defined in cultural terms just as many of the solutions must be in a cultural context. Because of the cultural aspect, the usefulness of combining crisis intervention and indigenous paraprofessional workers is apparent. In any event, working in crisis situations may often involve several therapists and interveners at various levels of training and from a variety of disciplines.

While the goals of crisis intervention are to stabilize and to get the person back to the person's point of functioning before the crisis occurred, the means of doing so in crisis intervention can and do vary widely. Flexibility is probably the best way of describing the therapist's approach. It can range from support and catharsis to direct instructions or visits to the family or the community as is indicated and necessary.

As more and more experience with the crisis approach accumulates, probably more accurate descriptions of the techniques and the method will be possible. At this time it seems to be a means of providing fast and effective help in emergency situations and to be a prime means of helping those from lower socioeconomic situations.

Suicidal crisis

There are probably few if any people who have not at some time during their lives thought of or considered committing suicide. People under emotional stress and undergoing difficulties in their lives of the kind that lead to crisis situations are more prone to suicide thoughts and impulses than are others. Many people presenting crisis problem situations may often also have suicide thoughts or have made a suicide attempt. In dealing with people in crisis, the therapist must be alert to suicidal concerns that may be a part of many other crisis situations.

Suicidal thoughts and behaviors are, however, not always limited to crisis situations. It is necessary for the crisis therapist to be aware of the risk factors and the behaviors that indicate potential suicidal individuals. Once the suicidal potential has been established, intervention measures must be started without delay.

Assessing suicide potential—risk factors

Suicidal thoughts and intentions often occur or are associated with depression. A mood state of sadness with feelings of guilt and a sense of inadequacy and hoplessness are often present. Other signs that may indicate depression are recent weight loss, loss of appetite, sleeplessness, fatigue, and sexual impotence or loss of sexual desire. Depression, along with anger and agitation, especially when it has come on suddenly, is a matter for particular concern in a person who has indicated suicidal potential. However, it must be noted that some individuals may be suicidal even though the depressive indications are not present.

When suicide is a concern, the crisis therapist must make a rapid emergency evaluation of an individual's suicidal potential. In order to do so, the therapist must establish communication with the patient in order to get the patient to bring out troubled feelings. The suicide threat or attempt is often viewed as the patient's cry for help. The crisis worker must recognize these behaviors as pleas for help and provide help. Suicidal individuals are most likely to kill themselves when they are no longer in communication with others. But often they have communicated many earlier indications about their intent. Some clues to suicidal intent are statements like, "I'm tired of living—soon I won't be around," or "My family would be better off without me." Those who are most seriously suicidal generally have strong feelings of hopelessness, exhaustion, and failure and those who "just want out."

Another combination of factors that has been found especially lethal is severe depression in association with psychotic thinking or with alcoholism or drunkenness and confusion.

There are several other important factors that have been associated with a high degree of suicidal risk. They are discussed in the following paragraphs.

The age and sex of the individual must be considered. Males are much more likely to complete suicide than are females, and the older the individual, generally the more serious the suicidal potential. The danger of killing oneself increases with age for white males. White males over age fifty who are communicating suicidal thoughts should always be taken very seriously. Adolescence is also a high peak risk age, especially for certain ethnic minority males, Indians and Eskimos, for example.

Females from age fifteen to thirty-five make the largest number of nonlethal suicide attempts. These attempts seem generally more to influence another person's behavior than a wish to die. It is also true that females choose less violent methods in their attempts than do men; furthermore, women usually are much more willing to communicate their concerns and to seek help.

Generally, the more sudden and acute the onset of the suicidal crisis, the greater the immediate danger of a completed suicide. If there have been recent attempts or if there has been an extensive pattern of previous attempts, these, too, are danger signals of lethality. It is not true that those who talk about suicide or have made previous attempts will not do it. But in the long run, those who have the acute, sudden onsets have the best prognosis for making a good adjustment when they come out of the crisis period. Those who have had long-standing repeated depressive episodes and suicidal concerns even without the sudden onset have an increased likelihood of completing suicide sometime in the future as they grow older.

Whether or not the individual has made a specific choice of method, time, and place for the suicide is another key indicator. It is a very serious sign if the individual has. The choice of a method of great lethality, such as a gun or jumping from a high place, is also a very dangerous indication. The ingestion of certain fast-acting drugs should also be considered a situation of great danger.

Another indicator of seriousness is when the suicidal person has suffered a recent loss of a loved one through whatever means, such as death or separation or divorce. When the loss is a permanent one, this factor is of even more significance and danger.

Another such sign is when there has been a recent severe illness or hospitalization, especially in older people. Then the likelihood of a serious suicide attempt is increased.

An evaluation of the resources available to the patient is crucial. The attitude of the husband or wife, the relatives, or friends makes a great difference. If the others are helping and interested, these are positive indicators. If the others are rejecting or don't care, this is an indicator of a negative outcome.

Some additional factors associated with how lethal a suicidal person might be have to do with whether or not the suicidal person has any sort of permanent relationships with others. People who have very unstable relationships, have alcoholism problems, are impulsive, and portray a sense of being emotionally burnt out are high-risk individuals. Considerable disorganization of the person's thinking and feelings to the extent that he or she can no longer reason realistically or cope adequately with his or her environment is another negative indicator.

Was it a suicide?

What is a suicide is not always clear. In terms of the reported statistics on suicide, it is very likely that suicide is underreported. Because of the stigma surrounding suicide, there is great pressure on physicians and others to certify such deaths as natural or accidental. Families do not want the deaths recorded as suicide. In addition, in approximately 75 percent of the cases, insurance money may not be paid in full for a suicidal death.

The *psychological autopsy* is a method that has been developed to investigate uncertain cases. As has been indicated before, suicidal persons often leave many clues to their intentions days or weeks before they kill themselves. The psychological autopsy attempts to determine the individual's state of mind prior to the death by investigating the individual's activities and by interviewing people with whom the victim was very close and would know the individual's most recent behavior. The questions focus on such issues as: Did the person intend to die during his or her last days of life? Was the person depressed? Had the person seen a physician prior to death? Had the person spoken as if he or she were suicidal?

Sometimes, however, what appears to be a suicide might more accurately be an accident. An autopsy can help establish this for the family.

There are many cases which, while not clearly suicidal, nonetheless, have some of the elements of suicide. These have been called *subintended deaths*. There are many apparent accidents or even natural deaths that have a considerable element of a subintended wish to die. For instance, some people may want to die but will not act consciously on it. Rather, they live carelessly and may unconsciously imperil their lives. For instance, the chronically ill person may stop taking the necessary medicine. A depressed person may drive very fast and recklessly. Still other cases have been known in which individuals actually taunt and tempt someone else to kill them. Russian roulette, one-car accidents, and taking unneeded risks may fall in this category. Because of these sub-intended deaths, the established suicide rates are probably lower than they actually are.

Sometimes, of course, the opposite occurs. An individual who does not intend to die uses the suicide attempt as a means of trying to influence another person. But the individual misjudges the situation. The intended rescuer doesn't come to the rescue in time and the victim unintentionally dies. An example is that of a woman who turned on the gas and put her head in the oven several minutes before her husband usually came home from work. That particular day he was late and she died.

Coping with a person in a suicidal crisis

The basic steps in dealing with a suicidal emergency are to (1) establish a relationship with the suicidal individual and maintain the contact in order to obtain the essential information to assess the lethality; (2) identify and clarify what the recent stress is the individual is reacting to, along with finding out the individual's circumstances and basic problem; (3) evaluate the lethality of the suicide potential by thoroughly considering the factors of age, sex, suicide plan, stress, depressive symptoms, resources, lifestyle, communication, medical condition, and the reactions of significant others in the person's life; (4) assess what strengths and resources are available to the individual and mobilize them to provide maximal help; and (5) develop a therapy plan and take appropriate action. If, for instance, the acute suicidal behavior is not appreciably reduced as a result of initial contact, steps may have to be taken to have the individual closely watched or hospitalized. When the suicidal intent can be sufficiently reduced or when the evaluation indicates that it is not critically lethal, the plan for mobilization of available resources can be implemented by using the initial contact information, including the developed relationship. Arrangements for continuing the contact and for carrying out the therapeutic plan must be diligently followed up.

Preventive actions

Educational programs that focus on helping people to recognize suicidal feelings and the indications of self-harm intentions in themselves and in others are useful. Such programs teach the early warning signs of suicide intent and alert people to the cry for help. Equally important is education to remove the stigma of suicide so that suicide can be openly talked about and dealt with. If people feel free to come for help early, they may not reach the more serious and deadly stage.

When there has been a completed suicide, the dead person is not the only victim. The family or those intimately involved with the deceased are also victims. Often they are neglected, but they need continuing support and emotional assistance for their loss, and perhaps for their feelings of guilt. In addition, they may feel shame and will likely feel stigmatized. The children, especially the young children of the suicidal parent, are in some ways more the victim than the one who committed suicide.

Suicide attempts must be followed up, for eight out of ten people who do successfully kill themselves have attempted suicide before. Therefore, suicide attempts should always be taken seriously. Even when the crisis is past, it is important to have a follow-up. Determining how deadly the intention is is not always easy, but the intention is really more important than the method.

Suicide prevention centers that provide available walk-in or telephone contact are among the best resources for suicide prevention. They can be manned by trained volunteers from the community who have professional consultation available. Communities that have unusually high rates of suicide should certainly develop them. Such a crisis facility is an important and necessary resource in any community.

summary

1 Crisis intervention as therapy is the means of choice for acute situational disturbances. A crisis is an urgent emergency situation that could have a disastrous outcome. Developmental crisis refers to situations associated with developmental stages such as adolescence or aging, accidental crises to life events such as experiencing loss through the death of someone close.

2 People in crises experience great stress and are usually open to receiving help. Crisis intervention has been especially useful for people of lower socioeconomic status who otherwise would not avail themselves of mental health treatment. The stages of crisis are: extensive stress with which the person tries to deal by using previous methods, failing that greater disorganization, then seeking help and control, and failing that extensive disorganization.

3 Crisis intervention can be environmental manipulation, general support, or brief therapy to help the person understand his or her role in the problem situation. Crisis therapy involves helping the person maximize his or her own resources and develop self-understanding.

4 The crisis therapist must be flexible, warm, understanding, very active, and directive, must convey hope, confidence, and trust, and must rapidly assess the situation and the strengths and weaknesses of the patient and come up with a workable plan. The goal of crisis work is to stabilize the patient and get the patient back to the level of functioning before the crisis.

5 When the crisis includes the potential of suicide, special assessment of risk and special intervention methods are called for. Rapid evaluation of lethality includes assessing the strength of intent to commit suicide, the depth of depression, and the attitude of having given up. High-risk factors include male sex, middle age and older, or adolescence, sudden onset, previous attempts, definite plan, and lethal method.

6 Establishing a relationship with the suicidal person, assessing lethality, strengths, and resources, mobilizing resources, and developing a treatment plan or taking effective action are the main steps in dealing with a suicide crisis.

7 Prevention of suicide is promoted through educational programs to help people recognize the warning signs of suicide and by reducing the stigma so that people can seek early help. Prevention centers and telephone hotlines are especially useful.

Marital and family treatment methods

Humans are social animals and have as their primary natural social group their families. The basic unit of the family is usually the marital couple, but there are many single-parent families, and when this is the case, usually the parent is the mother. There are still other families which center around the grandmother or some broader extended family arrangement.

Families and marital couples are basic social units in all cultures and societies. Psychological difficulties are almost always closely tied into family and marital relationships. In many cases, treating just the individual is likely to be ineffectual because the problem lies in the family interactions or marital situations. Until that is worked out, little headway can be made working with the individual separately.

Generally speaking, marital therapy can be considered one form of family treatment. Marital therapy focuses on the interactions of the marital couple with each other; family therapy is mainly concerned with the relationships in the whole family unit. It is when the marriage is in trouble, when the partners do not get along, that marriage therapy is indicated. Family therapy, in some contrast to marital therapy, has a wider purpose: that of improving the functioning of the whole family as an interacting unit. Family therapy is the more recent method. It is usually used when one or more of the family members have been identified as having a serious personal adjustment problem that seems to have its basis in the family interactions and relationships. Rather than a single-family member being seen as a patient, the whole family group is considered the patient and the family is treated for the disorder as a unit, usually all together instead of separately.

Counseling marital problems

Marital difficulties or problems related to the marital relationship are among the most frequent problems that come to the attention of mental health services. The marital couple is the basic unit of the family, and the family is the basic unit of social organization of almost all peoples and cultures. Due to great social changes occurring throughout the world, traditional marital functions and relationships have undergone much change in almost all societies and cultures today. It is then not surprising that marriage which is the central, primary, social relationship would be very sensitive to social change. Indeed, the traditional marriage has suffered disruptions in many cultures. In Western industrialized societies, for instance, women have increasingly entered the job market and have gained more and more economic and social equality with men. The traditional need for the husband to be the provider and protector is much less crucial. Religious and legal restrictions on cohabiting relationships have been diminished. This has led to increasing numbers of young couples living together and producing children without legal or religious approval and without any commitment by the parents to stay with each other or be responsible for the offspring.

Among the economically disadvantaged and those societies emerging from a tribal organization the dominant position of the male has often been badly eroded. In these situations, unstable relationships between the marital couple often are fraught with physical violence and desertion by the male. Such families are essentially maintained and led by women.

As this pattern has become an increasingly frequent one, the number of couples that divorce or separate or have one or the other partner deserting seems to be constantly increasing. The price is often paid by the children. This is usually related to the long-standing conflict and instability of the adult relationship.

Marriage counseling defined

Marriage counseling is one form of family counseling, the one which concerns largely the interpersonal relationship of the marital couple. In its broadest view, it can also include the following: *premarital counseling*, which usually consists of helping the couple decide if they are suited enough to each other to be married as well as providing some guidance on how to get along; *predivorce counseling*, which involves working with a marriage that is in difficulty, either toward some solution to the problems and learning to live comfortably together or toward making the decision to divorce; *postdivorce counseling,* in which the focus is to work with the individuals to help with the adjustment of being single again; and *general family counseling,* which emphasizes the importance of the marriage to family living. Family counseling, in contrast to marital counseling, involves applying the general principles and techniques of counseling and psychotherapy for the purpose of dealing with the emotional conflicts and problem situations involved in a family difficulty. Originally, marriage counseling focused on each individual partner in separate counseling sessions on the assumption that the problem lay primarily in the separate individuals, but current practice now emphasizes the interactive relationship of the marital partners together. Counseling is usually now done in a conjoint interview that includes both partners of the marriage.

The counselor's role

As a general orientation, the marriage counselor must keep in mind not only the personalities of the two separate individuals involved but particularly the way they interact as partners. The counselor must consider each partner's feelings about himself or herself, each partner's view of the other partner, and what each expects of the other and themselves as a couple.

While some of the common causes of the immediate marital difficulty tend to be such factors as money, sexual maladjustment, children, infidelity, or the inlaws, often hidden in these situations is a more basic concern, the lack of sensitivity to the needs of one partner by the other. Thus, concern about the failure to consider the partner's feelings, the goals, values, and needs most often is more central than the other aspects.

Sex is, of course, a crucial part of a marital relationship, it being most often the initial basis of the attraction of the partners to each other. As a powerful source of need satisfaction, sex ultimately serves to bind the couple together in spite of all the differences, irritations, and difficulties of other interactions of living together. With the development of efficient birth control methods, effective treatments for venereal disease, and wide acceptance and availability of abortions, there has been a change toward much greater liberalization of sexual attitudes and behavior. At the same time as these changes have been taking place, there also have been great advances in the understanding of the actual functioning of human sexuality and effective methods have been developed for dealing with many types of sexual problem. Marriage counselors need to develop knowledge and skill in the area of sex therapy.

Types of marital involvement and implications for treatment

One way of conceptualizing marriage is in terms of the amount of personal relationship or involvement that the partners have with each other. This can range from very slight involvement at one extreme to a very full, rich relationship at the other as described by Mace (1972). It is mostly those marriages between the extremes, those that have some but not full involvement, that are most likely to have difficulty.

The utilitarian marriage—minimal relationship involved   The utilitarian marriage is not uncommon and it may still be the traditional marriage arrangement in developing areas or with certain lower socioeconomic groups. Such a marriage is not started with the ideal that the couple live happily ever after. Rather, it is for the purpose of serving certain practical and important community social functions, especially those of continuing the family line and property. The partners probably have had little or no choice in picking who they would marry, and they often live with one of the parental families instead of setting up an independent home. Such marriages may work very well and meet the goals that are intended in such an arrangement. Children are born, the wife's role is to care for the home and her husband's comfort, and he in turn provides her and the children with protection and security. When such marriages occur in situations where the traditional culture is no longer strong and the marriage is no longer closely watched over by the older generation, the arrangement then usually is in the form of a mutually acceptable bargain whereby each partner provides certain services for the other. Problems in this kind of marriage situation often take the form of family violence; the husband batters his wife or the husband fails to provide for his family. Neglect of the home and the children or infidelity is more likely to be the central form of problem behavior for the wife. Counseling for such relationships usually is done as crisis intervention or environmental manipulation. The therapist works toward helping the couple obtain needed legal assistance or return to the previous level of marital adjustment.

Marriages of partial relationship   Most marriages involve limited and restricted relationships. The couple begins the marriage with expectations that it will not only be a practical and useful arrangement but that it will also be for each of them a relationship of pleasure and mutual personal fulfillment. The duties in this kind of marriage are not different from those of the utilitarian marriage, but the roles are not so clearly determined. The primary orientation of each partner in this marriage is the hope for satisfaction and fulfillment from the relationship of a shared life. It is when they are not achieved that the couple becomes increasingly disenchanted. Often such marriages end in separation or divorce. Much of the problem is that the romantic ideal was unrealistic to begin with. It most likely was a fantasy on the part of each of the partners that was never fully shared or discussed with the other. Under such circumstances, it is very likely that there will be disappointments because each partner does not know, let alone live up to, the other's romantic expectations. These issues cannot be discussed and cannot be resolved. Instead, that part of the relationship becomes blocked off between the two of them. The result is an increasingly narrow relationship in the marriage. Some couples are willing to live together in such a very restricted and tenuous relationship, but others are not and at this point move to find grounds for dissolving the marriage. Others, however, may seek some help at this stage.

The full and satisfying relationship marriage   Marriages in which a really close, fulfilling, and satisfying relationship between the partners is developed and sustained are probably relatively rare. It has been estimated that less than 10 percent of marriages ever achieve such a full, rich relationship level. Furthermore, such marriage relationships do not happen instantly; the couples must develop them over a long period of time. It has been suggested that it may take at least 30 years to gain a really full, rich marriage relationship. In order for such a full relationship to develop, the partners must be mature people and have much sensitivity and consideration for each other. And more importantly, from the very beginning they must have very much in common with each other in terms of mutual values, goals, and interests. Such a relationship develops trust and unity, not from avoiding arguments or disagreements but rather from facing and working through interpersonal conflicts when they arise. Needless to say, these couples are rarely seen in marriage counseling. Those doing marriage counseling, nonetheless, could learn a great deal about what to aim for from observing and understanding such full relationship involvement marriages.

Key elements of marital relationship

Communication   The most basic part of the marital relationship is communication. Almost all of the marital problems seen by counselors have in large measure to do with misunderstandings, misinterpretations, and the resulting distrust between the partners because of the lack of clear communication with each other. It is not usually that they lack the ability to communicate. Rather, it is an unwillingness to do so on the part of one or both. When a relationship does not have full communication and mutual trust, living as closely together as in a marriage is bound to create very difficult problems. Lack of communication, or misleading or dishonest communication, or poor understanding soon leads to suspicion and resentment.

The fear of open and full communication is very often the result of a greater underlying fear that if one partner were to reveal his or her true thoughts and feelings, he or she would surely be disliked and rejected. The burden of effective communication is a two-way street. It is the responsibility of both the one who communicates and of the one to whom the message is addressed. This is so because how the message is received can either encourage and improve communication or can stifle or cut it off. The one who receives the message must be receptive and able to accept, understand, and tolerate a wide range of communications. Regularly responding to one's partner with ridicule, anger, rejection, or even worse, disinterest is the best way to break off the communication and to maintain a lack of communication.

It should be kept in mind that there are many ways of communicating without using words. The sexual relationship, among other things, is itself an important way in which the partners communicate with each other. The male who seeks only orgasmic release communicates to his wife that he has little regard for her feelings and her needs. The wife who submits as to an unpleasant duty conveys her lack of concern, interest, and caring to her husband. Sexual dysfunctions that interfere with full sexual performance to an even greater extent communicate interpersonal messages between the couple.

Sharing   Sharing is the next most important part of a marriage relationship. This has to do with the sharing of not only material possessions such as money and cars, but even more importantly, with the sharing of beliefs, hopes, ambitions, values, and behavioral standards. When people do not share values for the same things, they don't have the same aims and goals, and without those it is very difficult to develop a very full and meaningful relationship.

Sharing includes the sharing of relatives and friends. For a full sharing relationship, each partner's family must be accepted as the partner's own family, and they must have mutual friends.

Without a doubt, money is almost always the most sensitive test of the sharing part of the relationship. Agreeing on how limited financial resources will be spent and on who will be in charge of the spending is a very crucial aspect of compatibility in the area of money sharing.

The sharing of children is equally an important consideration in relationships. Sharing includes not only the responsibility, the effort, and work involved in caring for, disciplining, and providing for children but also the sharing of relationship bonds of each partner to the children with the other partner. It often happens that the battleground between couples is competition for the children's love. One partner may try to have one or more of the children relate more closely to him or her than to the other parent or may even try to turn them against the other parent.

Cooperation   A third important area in developing a very full marital relationship is that of cooperation. In a close relationship a couple not only needs to communicate and to share but also to work cooperatively together in all the important phases of the business of living together. Working together is needed in the running and the management of the home, in the caring for the children, in the family social and recreational activities, and in money arrangements and buying. Mutual planning for both immediate and future activities is necessary as well, for without planning much confusion can result. When there is a lack of agreement on future goals, there will likely be serious friction and conflict.

Some reasons why marriages fail

Perhaps the main reasons that many marriages run into trouble is that neither partner has much of an idea or understanding of how important the marriage relationship is, let alone know how to achieve it. It is very likely that most people have had little, if any, modeling of a good relationship from their own parents. They do not know what a good relationship should be. Even when the parents' relationship has been a good one, much of the closeness and sharing is usually hidden from the children. It is important that couples know why a good relationship is necessary and crucial, but very few have had the opportunity to know what a good model marriage is like in real life.

There are probably many people who go into marriage deliberately seeking only a very limited relationship. Men in particular in our society may have been raised with the idea that the male role requires being very independent and self-sufficient and that any needs for dependency must be denied. Such a person may deliberately stay away from a close relationship with anyone. For others, there is a fear that a close relationship will so restrict them that they will lose their freedom and autonomy to act and do things the way they want.

Another and perhaps the most difficult hindrance to a close relationship in a marriage is found in people who because of earlier experiences have developed severe psychological inhibitions to being open and fully able to be close. In this case, it usually is not possible to work it out in just the conjoint therapy with the couple and the counselor. Rather, such a situation may require more in-depth individual therapy for the partner who has such a severe problem.

Some basic aspects of interpersonal relationships

With the possible exception of the purely utilitarian marriage, it is generally the case that the quality of the relationship between the couple is the basic factor that will decide the satisfaction and success of the marriage. Below are listed some general qualities of relationships based on Adams' (1972) nine principles of interpersonal relationships. Being aware of these can be helpful in counseling couples whose relationship problems are the basis of the difficulty.

1. Relationships need time in which to grow and develop; they do not suddenly appear in full bloom after just a few interactions. In order to grow and prosper, a relationship requires that effort, time, and feeling be put into it. A relationship, even a well-developed one, will shrink and die unless time and effort are continually put forth to renew and refresh it. But it is also true that a relationship really cannot be forced and it cannot be developed by dishonest or selfish means or by one person alone. Time and effort are important to a relationship. Both parties must give in order to receive in any kind of meaningful and lasting relationship. In order to develop and maintain relationships, communications and interactions must be honest and direct by both parties.

2. It is important to recognize that the need for closeness and intensity of a relationship is different in different people. It is also different in the same person from time to time. But one individual can only deal with a very limited number of close, intense relationships at the same time.

3. While having relationships is very important, persons in a relationship must also maintain their personal sense of individuality and some areas of privacy.

This means that a relationship should not be so overpowering as to submerge one or both partners. Each partner in the relationship needs to maintain himself or herself as a separate, independent person, while at the same time still being deeply and intimately involved in the relationship with the other partner. There are many times when each partner of the marriage must deal separately and independently with some part of his or her life or situation. To be so totally involved with another person that an individual cannot respond as an independent person means that the individual probably cannot respond adequately to many situations. In addition, there can be many dangers to being fully submerged in a relationship. The danger of being totally dependent on the other member of the relationship and the danger of being so involved that the personal qualities that attracted the partner to the relationship to begin with are lost are two prime examples. Paradoxically, to maintain good relationships, people need to continue to develop themselves and their own interests. Through this means one can bring fresh enrichment to the relationship that a total involvement with another person would not permit. Total togetherness can indeed result in an oppressive and deadening effect in a relationship.

4. How involved and deep a relationship should be is best decided by mutual agreement between the partners. Each should be free to determine how extensive the relationship should be and how far it should go. Basically, this should be considered in terms of their concept of socially determined roles in the marriage and how they view the social expectations of their culture with regard to the nature and depth of the relationship. Couples have the option to decide if they wish to follow the culturally defined roles or if they want to redefine and create a new relationship role for themselves. For example, the male does not always have to be the aggressor or instigator of sex and the woman does not have to be a passive participant. Similarly, the couple can determine what role in the relationship each will take and to what extent each will wish to pursue it in caring for the house or providing economic support for the family, and so forth.

5. A really close interpersonal relationship is also characterized by such factors as mutual respect, trust, and communication. In addition, it includes the ability to understand how the other partner feels, the desire to reach out and involve the partner, and the sharing of aims and goals while still maintaining one's individuality and capacity for self-direction and self-control. These are, of course, ideals of what a good relationship should be. They can be approached, but they are not often easily obtained. It is useful to keep them in mind when evaluating the difficulties of marital couples since they can point to areas that are most in need of change.

6. The extent to which the partners are involved in relationships with other people is an important factor in how much satisfaction they need from the marital relationship. If each has other ongoing relationships in addition to the marriage, such as those

occurring in connection with employment, friends, and hobbies, there will be less of a need to seek satisfactions in the marriage. But if one partner has few relationships outside the marriage and the other partner has many other relationships, the imbalance will likely create a potentially difficult situation.

7. Marriage counselors need to be aware that a very poor relationship is usually difficult to change once it has become an established pattern. When a relationship is dead, it isn't realistic to think it can be revived. Counselors must face facts about what they can or cannot realistically accomplish.

8. In order for a relationship to change, both parties must want to change. There must be a change in their attitudes about themselves, their partners, and their situations. As is true with most clinical situations in which there is motivation for positive change, there is a good possibility of having a positive change take place. When a serious desire to change is not present, the chances for improvement are all but absent. A crisis situation sometimes may activate a couple's awareness of the need and desire to change, and it can serve as the point to start working out problems.

9. Relationships between people never remain fixed in the same place. They are constantly changing, evolving, expanding, growing, or shrinking as people's situations change. Thus, there must be flexibility in relationships to adapt to changes in the individuals concerned and to their changing circumstances, to their changing stages of life, and to other factors. When relationships don't grow and adapt to new circumstances, in some cases they may be better ended.

10. The sexual part of the relationship is usually a good indicator of how satisfactory the overall marital relationship is. When the marriage is going well, the sexual relationship usually is also mutually satisfying. When the overall relationship in the marriage is not good, the sexual relationship very likely is also unsatisfactory.

Methods of marriage counseling

The relationship, the couple's interpersonal linkage, is probably the basic factor that will determine whether or not a marriage relationship will be successful. Consequently, counseling methods must be primarily directed to the relationship through seeing the couple together interacting and relating. Although there may be certain exceptions to this approach in which separate partners are seen individually, the main focus, nonetheless, should be on the relationship and the interaction between the partners. This ordinarily can best be worked on in conjoint therapy sessions in which both partners are present. Establishing which areas are presenting the difficulty in the relationship is the basic first task for both the couple and the counselor. Evaluating the motivation level and desire to work out the problem to effect change is a very necessary part of the assessment that must be made in the opening phases of marital counseling.

When it has been determined jointly with the couple what the areas of conflict are and that the couple is really motivated to work on the problem toward a change, then appropriate counseling approaches can begin.

There is no one best method; what method is used depends on the problem and people involved, as well as on the skill, experience, and orientation of the counselor. Very directive and behavioral techniques are appropriate and effective for some situations, but relationship awareness and action-oriented methods are appropriate and effective for others. Instructional and practice methods may be useful, and so can the methods that involve developing self-awareness and feeling and understanding the needs of the other.

For certain marital situations, especially those that fall in the category of utilitarian marriage, more crisis-oriented methods and procedures are often most effective. For those situations in which the couple feels the lack of a close emotional relationship and satisfaction, finding the areas where the closeness is missing and developing communication between the partners is the approach. Better self-understanding, developing skills of sharing, and cooperating should all be systematically included in this approach to treatment.

Many mental health problems are at least partially an aspect of marital difficulty. Effective marriage counseling and therapy can often be seen as a primary prevention measure against severe emotional problems, as well as treatment for an immediate problem. For from marital discord stems frustrations, anger, and feelings of rejection, to name a few. Further, the mental health of the children often suffers when the parents do not get along.

An additional point must be added. In recent times there have been great social changes. Traditions, both social and religious, have been in many ways greatly weakened or even abandoned. As a consequence, deciding what is or is not a marriage is often a very difficult task. For mental health purposes, a workable definition of marriage is a stable sexual living together arrangement between two people. From this standpoint, it is not necessary to have legal or religious acceptance of the relationship, and it is not necessary that it be a heterosexual relationship. What has been said about the heterosexual marriage, relationship, and interaction basically applies to homosexual relationships as well. The need for counseling for homosexual couples is probably as great as it is for heterosexual couples.

Family therapy

The beginnings of family therapy

Psychotherapy was first developed as a way to treat individuals singly. The development of group therapy followed soon afterward, and it has been particularly useful in helping individuals who have trouble socializing. The central importance of the whole family's behavior when treating children was the crucial factor in the development of family therapy as a separate form of group therapy. This followed the increasing recognition that when the child was disturbed it was not just a problem within the child, but it also involved the family and social environment. From this standpoint, it then follows that treatment must include and involve the basic social environment in which the patient lives.

While family therapy is a form of group therapy, in several ways it is a very different form of group therapy. One very important difference between the usual group therapy and family therapy is that family members have a sometimes lengthy previous relationship and interaction among them but members of a group do not. Family members also have a continuing future together whether they are in therapy or not, but group members ordinarily have no further relationship once the group therapy is over. Also, family members interact with each other much of the time outside the group, but group members are involved with each other only at the group sessions. Some additional differences are that the family is a natural social and legal group of people, but therapy groups are in one way or another arbitrary. The family has a developed, formed set of roles and ways of interacting with each other, but group members form their roles and communication with each other as the group develops.

Findings from families of schizophrenics

Family therapy had another source of development: the investigations of the involvement and interactions of families in which one of the members had schizophrenia. The Palo Alto Research Group (Bateson, Jackson, Haley, & Weakland, 1956) started studying the communication patterns in families of schizophrenics and in 1956 developed the *double bind theory* of schizophrenia.

Similarly, Lidz (1963) studied the family patterns of a small number of schizophrenics and concluded that a primary aspect of the patient's developing schizophrenia was a pathological marital relationship between the patient's parents. In such families, according to Lidz, there is an unbalance in roles and domination, or a situation in which one or the other parent tries to alienate the child from the other parent.

Bowen (1959) came to a similar conclusion about the parental marital relationship in the families of schizophrenics.

To summarize these studies of families of schizophrenics and some others as well, the parents of schizophrenics are generally anxious, conflicted, and immature, and they do not cope with their own feelings very well. In these families the parents have a poor marital relationship, and the roles of the family members are generally fixed and inflexible. There seems to be much disturbance in relationships in such families. But still the child who eventually becomes schizophrenic may well have had some special impairments to begin with, and the schizophrenia is not just due to the family situation. It also seems that there is an interacting process going on between the parent and child in such situations and that the child also contributes to the family disturbance.

Studies stemming from family therapy have shown that the difficulty in family relationships often may only become apparent when the family members are directly observed together, rather than from usual clinical histories. Schizophrenia does not appear to develop simply as a function of a certain kind of mother or father. Rather, it seems to be more a matter of the relationship and interaction of the parents with each other. In addition, when observed as part of the family unit, the one who is schizophrenic plays a significant part in others' responses to him or her. The conclusion from this is that since these pathological family patterns may play a causal role in the development of schizophrenia, the treatment then should aim toward changing the pathological family interactional relationships.

Types of family therapy

Several forms of family therapy have been developed. In *conjoint* family therapy family members are seen at the same time and with the identified patient present. Sometimes the approach to treatment includes having all family members at the treatment session with the therapist. Other times the session does not include everybody, but rather various combinations of family members. The crucial thing about this method is that it seeks to understand the family as a total interacting group. But since some members of the family group are more likely to work well in treatment and others are not, it may be necessary to focus more on those members than on the others.

Assessing families for therapy

As is true for other treatment methods, family therapy also requires an evaluation of the problem situation or of the relationships within the family in order to develop effective goals and an appropriate treatment plan and to find effective means for improving the family situation. A variety of new approaches to the assessment of the family have been developed. These come partly from the research on family factors that might relate to the causes of schizophrenia.

In the more traditional assessment method separate evaluations of individual family members through interviews are made and sometimes psychological testing is done. However, from the standpoint of family therapy, the family is more than the sum of its individual members. The family as a group is considered a unique social unit in and of itself. To be really meaningful, the assessment must consider the total group interactions as a whole instead of the single assessment of each member.

Since there are different positions on the nature of family interactions, no one method of assessment is generally accepted. Assessment in any event introduces an observer and often an artificial situation, reaction to which may not indicate typical behavior, and thus not adequately represent the family. Nevertheless, adequate assessment is basic to effective treatment and must be made.

Interview methods of family assessment

Unstructured interviews Following clinical tradition, unstructured interviews with the family as a group and with individual family members is the most usual approach. The purpose of these interviews is generally to evaluate the family's strengths and weaknesses, its style of interrelating, and to determine goals and whether or not family therapy is an appropriate approach. In such interviews observations of behavior and interactions, traditional history, and each family member's view of the situation are considered. Assessment and the beginning point of therapy proceed simultaneously. Assessment and therapy often best proceed as a simultaneous process.

Structured interviews There are certain disadvantages to the traditional unstructured, free-ranging clinical interviews, and several methods have been devised to remedy the situation. One approach is to give family members as a group some individual or joint problem and observe their interactions while dealing with it. The *Wiltwyck Family Task* method has eight activities for the family to do as a group. The activities are presented by standard, tape-recorded instructions and the assessors watch through a one-way vision screen in order not to interfere with the family interaction. The activities that family members are asked to do are:

1. Agree on a meal that everyone would like.

2. Decide such things as which family member is the most bossy, which one causes the most trouble, which one gets away with the most, and which one is the cry baby.

3. Consider a family argument that happened at home and explain the way it started and how it came out.

4. Make a plan on how to spend a ten-dollar gift so that everybody will be satisfied.

5. Each member tell what things other family members do that pleases him or her and also what they do that displeases him or her.

6. Work together to assemble a small toy building.

In this procedure there are two further assessment problems:

1. The family is asked to choose one small gift from a group of things which include a group game, an individual game, and an age- or sex-specific game.

2. Refreshments are given to the family, but there is one cupcake and one drink less than needed for the group. How the family deals with this situation and their sharing pattern are observed.

Another somewhat similar method of structured family interview is that developed by the Mental Research Institute (MRI). This method has the advantage of being able to be completed in about an hour's time. It consists of five parts. In part one, the family members are asked privately and individually what they think the main family problems are. Then the family is brought together and told of the different views. The interaction and discussion of the family are observed. In part 2 the family is asked to plan some sort of family together project. Part 3 is done without the children. The parents are asked to describe and discuss how they met each other. In part 4 the parents are asked to figure out the meaning of a proverb, and then with the children back with them, teach the children the meaning of the proverb. In part 5 each family member writes down on a card what he or she thinks is the fault of the family member sitting at his or her left. The therapist adds some statements to what is written on each card and then each card is read to the group, which is asked to guess to whom does this description apply.

These structured, task-oriented interviews develop ongoing interactions among the family which might not be available from observations from simple discussions or from family reports. What is also useful is that the information brought out to the observers is also brought out to the family members. Such structured interviews really provide not only a place to start therapy but also an assessment method.

Psychological tests in assessment of family therapy

Projective tests, the kind that present a rather unclear picture or situation for the person to respond to, have been used in family therapy assessment in both traditional ways and recently in different and rather innovative ways. They are given to each individual for assessment in the standard form. However, in the family interaction or consensus forms the procedures are given to the family as a group to agree upon a response. The response which results from the family's agreed decision is the one that is considered and interpreted. Also, there have been attempts to develop special test stimuli about family relationship themes for this kind of consensus analysis of the family group as a whole. Along the same lines, even intelligence tests have been given and analyzed in this conjunct way. The family interaction in arriving at an answer is mainly the way such tests are used in the assessment. This has been described as a useful way for learning about what has been called family intelligence and decision making.

A number of other family evaluation methods have been described, but most of them have not been well worked out. Usually, they involve devising situations in which the family is supposed to solve a task, but actually a successful solution is not possible. How the family deals with the problem and the disagreements are what the evaluation aims to determine. A method called *unrevealed differences* is one in which each family member is asked to pick from a list of ten possibilities which they would most prefer, such as which famous people they might want to meet, what foods they would most like to order if they went out for dinner, which movies they would like to see, or places they would like to visit, and so forth. The amount and kinds of differences among the family members in these areas are shared and discussed in the family group.

Research has shown that in comparison to families that are considered normal, those that have a schizophrenic, delinquent, or maladjusted member are more likely to show more disagreement and conflict in the way they solve problems as a group or in how they share interests.

Theories of family disorders

Research on family relationships, especially studies that deal with families that are likely to have schizophrenic children, has formulated several theories on the kinds of family relationships that seem to produce the problem behavior.

The double bind hypothesis   Bateson, Jackson, Haley, & Weakland (1956) hypothesized that a major factor in the cause of schizophrenia was that the patient was put in an impossible dilemma situation by constant and powerful conflicting communications from one or the other parent. Responding to one set of instructions would automatically make the person wrong by the second instruction, and, similarly, responding to the second set of instructions would automatically make the person wrong by the first set of instructions. Such contradictory and conflicting messages in the typical double bind situation usually occur at two different levels of communication. One of the messages may be clear, open, and direct, telling the person to do a certain thing. The other message is indirect, not open, and almost secret, but, nonetheless, it clearly communicates a message that tells the person to do the thing the opposite way.

There must be certain conditions for a double bind to take effect. These include the following: (1) It requires an ongoing communication link between two or more people, one of whom becomes the victim who is double binded. (2) The double binding situation must occur frequently to the extent that the victim almost automatically expects it in the communication link. Receiving a few such double messages is ordinarily not sufficient to have great effect.

The basic double binding message that the victim receives is usually in the form of a restriction with the threat of punishment if it is not followed. For example, "Don't do such and such or you will be punished" or "If you do such and such, you'll be punished." This aspect of the double bind is thus based on avoiding punishment rather than on doing or not doing things because that would bring a reward.

The second part is that in addition to the basic message there is a second restriction that conflicts with the first restriction. This message usually is given in a more hidden, subtle form. It threatens punishment for carrying out the first message. This second message may be communicated more by nonverbal means—gestures, voice tone, and actions.

In order for the double bind to work, there must be another condition. The victim must be trapped in the situation and unable to get away from the conflicting demands. This is most likely to occur in the case of a young child who is very dependent on a mother who is giving the double messages.

The last part of double binding happens when the victim generalizes double binds to many other situations and usually expects them. At this stage, the victim can react to any aspect of the double bind conditions as if the entire process has happened to him or her.

An example might be that of a mother who has an overweight teenage daughter. The mother's openly stated message and instructions to the girl are that she should diet and that she would be scolded and shamed if she does not. But an opposite and disguised message is in the fact that the mother serves the daughter large portions, makes many rich, tempting foods, and implies that if the daughter doesn't eat everything that mother worked so hard to prepare, it means she is disrespectful and doesn't love her mother. Thus, the daughter is punished if she doesn't diet, but she also incurs punishment (loss of love of mother) if she refuses to eat the rich ample food prepared. Caught in such an impossible to win situation, the victim experiences frustration, anxiety, and the kind of stress that may lead to severe psychopathology.

This same general research has shown that double binding family interaction styles tend to become quite set and to be very difficult to change. It seems that when people interact over a long time, they develop set ways of relating to each other and these are maintained by unspoken rules. Once these rules are established, people seem to have great resistance either to breaking them or to allowing new ways of relating to become established. But a new pattern of relating is exactly what is needed in order to improve the pathological relationship patterns of these families.

The Lidz psychoanalytic view   Basically, Lidz' (1963) research indicates that the main problem in families is due to disturbed relationships between the parents and the children. From this point of view, in order to develop normal, psychologically healthy children, it is necessary for the parents to have a cooperative relationship through which appropriate sex roles and ways of coping with the environment can be consistently and systematically role modeled for the children.

There were two major pathological marital relationships found in these studies. These marriages were considered to be so disturbed that they would likely produce disturbed or even schizophrenic children. The *marital schism* relationship is one in which there is a long-standing situation of friction and disagreement between the parents. Characteristics of this marriage are frequent threats of separation, much arguing, and constant struggles over power but without any resolution. So it goes on and on. Such squabbling parents may seek to have the children on their side, doing this by blaming and devaluing the other parent. The child is trapped in the middle, put in a conflict situation about loyalty to one parent or to the other. Research has suggested that females are more vulnerable to developing schizophrenia than are males when raised in a parental marital schism family situation.

In the other main relationship pattern described by Lidz, called the *marital skew*, the marital relationship is characterized by the domination of one parent over the other. Most usually it occurs in the form of one parent's needs being satisfied at the expense of the other parent's needs. In this situation the dominant parent may form a too close relationship with one of the children and exclude the other parent or other children. Males raised in this type of family are considered to be most vulnerable to schizophrenia.

Other views   Other studies have pointed to the pathological different features in the family relationship that produces schizophrenia. These include the patterns of thinking and attention that parents display and teach the child, for example, parents whose behavior models shift, whose attention is unfocused, or whose reasoning is very disturbed or illogical. Similarly, problems develop when relationship patterns are fraught with inconsistency. An example would be a mother who relates with sudden closeness and then withdrawal from her husband or child. Such pathological patterns usually are associated with families in which there are strong feelings of helplessness and hopelessness. Another theory concerns a relationship pattern in which the mother and child never really become emotionally separate from each other. Still another theory identifies parents who live together but are emotionally separate. In this case, they may outwardly seem to be happily married, but in fact they have a very poor, empty relationship.

Goals and objectives of family therapy

Since much of family therapy has come from research on family involvement in the development of schizophrenia, it has been used very often as part of the treatment program of young hospitalized schizophrenics. But it is often used in connection with other family based problems as well. It is useful, for instance, in a case in which an adolescent needs to become separate from the family, or in which family difficulties involve emotional estrangements among the members, or in which family difficulties involve disturbed and poor communications or much emotional distancing among family members.

Some of the conditions needed in order for family therapy to be effective are: (1) There must be a real family unit whose members are emotionally concerned and tied with each other and really want to find some kind of help for their family problem. (2) A "good" therapist must be available. The same general characteristics described earlier for good clinical work apply to family therapy as well. Perhaps especially necessary are the therapist's characteristics of self-awareness, ability to take leadership and to limit certain behaviors, and capacity for self-restraint.

Often having a co-therapist of the opposite sex can improve the effectiveness of the treatment and focus the issues more clearly. The two therapists must understand each other's methods and must work together instead of competitively on the case.

In general, the main goal of family therapy is to strengthen the family as a group. This goal is attained by helping family members to improve their communication with each other. The therapist needs to be a positive role model for clear, direct, open communication. Further, the therapist points out the clear meanings and hidden messages in the communication among members by checking out what was said and then what was understood. The need for the family members to talk to each other openly rather than indirectly is stressed by the therapist. Practice in doing this is important. It is through the direct expression of what the family members really think and feel that they learn about themselves and what the others are really like.

It is generally the rule that the therapy work be done with the family as a group with all members being there. One particular member's problem should not be the focus often or for a very long period. If one member's problem requires much particular attention, that member should be seen separately as an individual treatment case.

The focus in family therapy is coping with the here-and-now interactions of family members, not emphasizing the past history of these problems, or even the motivations behind them. Instead of seeking an understanding of the roots of the problem, family therapy works more for direct action and change.

Another general goal of family treatment is to help family members not only increase their individuality and separateness but also maintain a place in the family unit. This is important because the more the members develop some mature individuality and freedom from overdependence on or domination from the family unit, the better they can relate to each other relevantly and on approximately equal terms. This makes for an effective functioning family group.

A third important goal is that of enhancing the marriage relationship of the parents. It is not unusual to find that when there is a family problem involving a child, there is also some difficulty in the marital relationship. When the marriage problem can be identified early and some improvement in the relationship can be made, there will likely be positive changes in the problems of other members of the family. When a definite marriage problem has been uncovered in the course of family treatment, it may be necessary to see the marital couple separately and focus treatment on a marital counseling procedure. (A more detailed discussion of marriage counseling was discussed earlier in this chapter.) If family therapy is still necessary, it is started again after some good progress has been made in the marital situation.

Techniques in family therapy

Family therapy is a form of group therapy, and many of the general methods and approaches of group therapy are properly used in the family therapy situation. There is, of course, no one approach to family therapy. Rather, each of the different approaches stresses different problem areas and uses its own special way for working with the family.

It is generally agreed, though, that the focus of family therapy is not just the marital couple, but rather the family as a unit itself. There are, however, some procedures used in working with the family in which focusing on individuals does occur. For instance, it is sometimes useful for the other family members to become acquainted with the feelings and difficulties of an individual member by bringing them out through individual therapy with that member during the family therapy session. Further, some forms of family therapy accept the position that some members of the family are much more amiable to working on problems than others. Here the focus of the treatment is on those who are workable and with whom there can be some effect. One technique is to have an individual family member develop the role of the family expert on how the family unit interacts and on how it might usefully change. This procedure is much like training a paraprofessional to provide help for his or her own family.

When communication is the problem within the family, the main emphasis should be on developing improved communication skills. An important part of this is learning how to listen to the other person and to try to understand that person's point of view. Techniques to help family members actually become aware of how they interact and how they behave are also very helpful. This can be done by having some family members observe the interaction of others and bring their observations to the therapy discussions. Other methods include such things as video tape playback of family sessions or the use of one-way vision mirrors to observe the rest of the family.

Some methods from behavior modification have been used in family therapy. One such procedure involves identifying and determining the frequency of unwanted behaviors and reactions and then rewarding the family members with recognition and approval for the behavior that is wanted. Role playing is also an effective technique. This is a method in which individuals may play the role of the person with whom they are having difficulty or may try new behavior under safe conditions.

In general, family therapy considers and uses techniques and methods from many of the other approaches to therapy. What the goals will be depends upon the theoretical orientation of the therapist.

In family therapy the therapist plays a very active part, always being alert to all interactions. The therapist must be firm, positive, and direct in maintaining the therapy course toward the goal. The therapist makes certain that therapeutic aims are being actively pursued by making sure that the focus is mostly on what the family as a unit is doing and not on individuals in the family.

summary

1 The family is the basic unit of society and the marital couple the basic unit of the family. Marital therapy focuses on the marital couple, and family therapy focuses on the total family unit. Marriage difficulties are frequently involved in mental health problems, particularly as a result of the changing roles of men and women and changes in views of sexuality.

2 Some marriages are utilitarian for the purpose of children, family life, and convenience. No romantic expectations are included. Most marriages are of partial relationships with expectations of fulfillment which are usually disappointing because of emotional constrictions. There are only a few marriages that are really full and satisfying.

3 The key elements for a successful marriage relationship are communication, sharing, and cooperation. Marriage fails when the partners do not understand the importance of the relationship, have no knowledge of how to achieve the relationship, or are unwilling to become so involved.

4 Some important basic aspects of relationships are that they need time to grow and constant attention to prosper. People differ in their need for closeness. People also need to maintain individuality and some areas of privacy. The depth of the relationship and the rules need to be mutually agreed upon. The extent of other relationships determine in part how great the need for the marital relationship. When poor relationships have reached a certain point, they probably cannot be revived. Both parties must want change if change is to take place. The relationship is always changing and individuals must adjust. The sexual relationship often is a good indicator of the overall relationship.

5 Marital counselors work usually with the couple to enhance the relationship in all aspects.

6 Family therapy views behavioral problems and disorders in terms of family interactions and treatment is based on that position. The emphasis is on the family as a group. While family therapy is usually started because of the problems of one family member who is identified as the patient, family therapists do not consider that any one family member is the patient.

7 A number of negative family patterns and interactions have been associated with the development of a schizophrenic individual in the family. These include communication and logical distortions in dealing with each other, maneuvering members into impossible double bind emotional conflicts, and various patterns of marital relationship difficulties.

8 The family therapy treatment approach is based on group therapy and uses techniques from many areas, but it focuses on improving communication, developing logical, reality-based expectations and stresses emotionally direct and honest interactions.

9 A number of innovative family tasks have been developed to help assess problem areas of family interactions.

10 The goal is effectively integrating the family unit, but it is paradoxical that one way to that end is to help the individual family members become realistically independent and separate while still remaining fully a part of the family group.

Problem drinking and alcoholism: Effects and treatment

Alcoholism, depending on how it is defined, is a disorder that affects directly over nine million people in the United States, and indirectly many more. It is a complex disorder with many social, personal, and physical consequences. While it is as yet poorly understood, there is no shortage of views about the cause and treatment (Tarter and Sugerman, 1976).

Alcohol, when drunk in small amounts, can have many pleasant and positive results. For instance, it can enhance such desirable things as relaxation, social comfort, and communication. But when drunk in large amounts over long periods, alcohol becomes a serious danger to both physical and psychological health. That type of drinking can result in dependence on or addiction to alcohol and can lead to severe social and personality deterioration that is very harmful to the individual's ability to function. That alcohol effects can vary from positive to destructive may be one of the main reasons why people generally have very mixed feelings about drinking. Drinking is considered to be all right, but drunken behavior is not acceptable. The positive effects are immediate and appealing, the negative effects come later. Often alcohols' destructive results are not apparent to many until it is too late.

Symptoms, causes, and concepts

Defining alcoholism

Defining alcoholism is difficult and complex. Regular drinking or even drunkenness is not behavior in and of itself sufficient to define alcoholism. This is partly due to the fact that patterns of drinking vary from country to country and are very culturally specific.

Jellinek (1946, 1962) has made some very important and useful observations that help to clarify drinking patterns and the concept of alcoholism. He distinguished between the addictive and the nonaddictive alcoholic. The crucial difference is in the loss of control in which the addictive alcoholic experiences a physical demand for alcohol and will continue to drink until too intoxicated or too sick to drink more. Jellinek pointed out that there are many patterns of drinking, not all of which are addictive or are necessarily alcoholism.

Jellinek developed his descriptions of phases and types of alcoholism from a survey of drinking behavior of Alcoholics Anonymous (AA) members. From his survey studies Jellinek describes phases of alcoholism. The *prealcoholic phase* begins socially. The individual gains marked relief from drinking and comes to use it for tension reduction. In the *prodromal phase* the drinker suffers sudden blackouts while drinking. In this phase the drinker is very concerned with alcohol, will gulp drinks, and feels guilty about his or her drinking behavior. In the *crucial phase* the frequency of blackouts increases and the individual loses complete control of the ability to refrain from drinking. Any drinking of alcohol may start a chain reaction in which the drinker feels an intense demand for continued alcohol. It is during this period that the drinker may find all kinds of excuses for his or her drinking behavior, and the drinker also may be very expansive about himself or herself, aggressive, or sometimes very sad. Further, during this period the only control is for the drinker to try periods of total abstinence from drink. Because of his or her behavior when drinking, in this phase the drinker may experience the loss of friends and/or jobs, sometimes family. In the *chronic phase* the drinker's behavior and relationships continue to deteriorate. The drinker may develop tremors and fears, have a noticeable decrease in sexual drive, and often become very jealous. Jellinek concluded that alcoholism is a complex and progressive disease in the physical sense.

Jellinek classified alcoholism into several types designated by Greek alphabet letters. *Alpha alcoholism* is a purely continued psychological reliance on alcohol to relieve tension. It doesn't lead to loss of control and it doesn't show signs of being a progressive process. In *beta alcoholism* there are physical complications from drinking such as gastritis or cirrhosis of the liver which may occur without physical or psychological dependence on alcohol.

Gamma alcholism is the predominating form in the United States and is most usually thought of as alcoholism. It involves: (1) increased physical tolerance to alcohol, (2) craving, (3) loss of control, and (4) withdrawal symptoms. This form often follows the phases of alcoholism described above.

Delta alcoholism is similar to gamma alcoholism except that the drinkers do not lose control but they are dependent on a certain amount of alcohol each day, but that amount does not increase. This is a pattern found frequently in France and wine-drinking countries.

Epsilon alcoholism is heavy episodic drinking bouts including "spree drinking" and "fiesta drinking." Jellinek points out that there are many other forms of alcoholism if alcoholism is defined as any drinking that causes damage to the person.

The physical disease concept of alcoholism became widely accepted. It certainly has been a much more positive way of looking at alcoholism than the previous view that alcoholic behavior was a form of moral degeneracy and deliberate evilness. But in the scientific field there is controversy and debate over whether or not alcoholism is a disease or a socially learned behavioral habit. This is complicated by the fact that there is considerable difficulty in precisely defining what constitutes alcoholism.

According to Alcoholics Anonymous, alcoholism is a disease which shows itself mainly by uncontrollable drinking. In this view, alcoholism can develop, if left untreated, into more and more serious physical and behavioral consequences. A heavy drinker is one who drinks by choice, but the alcoholic has no choice and no control. The alcoholic ends up drinking against his or her own will and desire. Alcoholics Anonymous believes that the disease of alcoholism can be held in check, but that alcoholics always remain alcoholics and cannot drink again without also restarting the disease process.

There are other much broader definitions of alcoholism that have been recently proposed. Keller and Efron (1955) have defined it as "characterized by repeated drinking that interferes with the drinker's health or social functioning." Keller has refined that definition further: "Alcoholism is repeated implicative drinking of alcoholic beverages so as to cause injury to the drinker's health or social and economic functioning." Other characteristics that have been considered to indicate alcoholism are: drinking secretively, rationalizing reasons for drinking, gulping drinks, and importantly, loss of control over drinking.

The criterion for alcoholism by the National Council on Alcoholism includes three levels: (1) classical symptoms such as gross tremors, hallucinations, withdrawal symptoms, or delirium tremens (DTs); (2)

symptoms of physical diseases which are often associated with alcoholism, such as alcoholic hepatitis, liver cirrhosis, and so forth; (3) behaviors often associated with alcoholism such as employment that facilitates drinking, frequent automobile accidents, or family disruptions.

Another definition of alcoholism is the modified definition of the World Health Organization. In WHO's view, alcoholics are those excessive drinkers whose dependence on alcohol has reached such a degree that they show a noticeable mental disturbance or an interference with bodily and mental health, interpersonal relationships, and social and economic functioning or they show the impending signs of such developments. They therefore require treatment, with the implication of this being that alcoholics have an illness.

The reason for so many definitions of alcoholism has to do with the fact that there is no one pattern that fits all situations. Jellinek's description of the progressive deterioration pattern (gamma alcoholism) is probably most widely known. His definition requires that the classical attributes of physical addiction be present, that is, the craving and increased tolerance for alcohol—needing more and more over time in order to have the effect—and the physical withdrawal symptoms upon stopping.

However, there are drinkers who cause society or themselves harm but do not show the classical craving for alcohol, or the increased need for more and more alcohol, or the physical withdrawal symptoms of drug dependency. The opposite pattern is not infrequently found. Some people become dependent on alcohol, but they do not seem to experience at least immediate social or personal harm from the alcohol. Further, drinking patterns vary from culture to culture. Episodic binge drinking is frequently noted among certain American Indian groups and others who often seem capable of stopping, often apparently without withdrawal symptoms. There is the so-called French drinking pattern in which there is a dependency on a regular fixed amount of alcohol drunk daily, but increased tolerance does not seem to occur.

The broad definition of Davies (1976) avoids some of the pitfalls of other definitions. His definition is: "Intermittent or continued use of alcohol associated with dependency (psychological or physiological) or harm in the sphere of mental, physical, or social activity." This definition covers situations of individuals who may not be continuous drinkers, those who are dependent on the drug and yet are experiencing no harm from it, and those who are experiencing harm but are not dependent on the drug. Such a definition is useful since there is much evidence to suggest that many individuals drink with the result of causing themselves and society much harm but do not show signs of drug dependency such as craving and increased tolerance. The opposite situation also occurs. There are many whose drinking does not cause social and immediate personal harm, but they do in fact show drug dependency. Therefore, this broader definition seems more meaningful and to more fully represent the various situations that seem to fall under the concept of harmful drinking.

Approaches to causes of alcoholism

The causes and the developmental course of alcoholism are really poorly understood. There are, however, no lack of proposed explanations, most of which can muster some supporting evidence, but no one approach can effectively explain more than a small segment of the problem in any effective way.

The moral model   The moral model of alcoholism has been around probably the longest and is of historical interest. It comes from religious and philosophical views with regard to excessive drinking. From this point of view, people who drink to the degree of going beyond what is acceptable in their culture are considered to be basically immoral. They are considered to be deliberate abusers who choose to indulge their own pleasures and refuse to control themselves. Thus from this standpoint, alcoholics are responsible for their own troubles, since they are considered to be deliberately indulging themselves. Therefore, they deserve to suffer the consequences of their behavior, both psychological and physical.

This attitude is still very much around today although in somewhat different form. Alcoholics Anonymous implies that there is a kind of moral lack in the problem drinker, and a change in the style of life by remaining dry and by making restitution to those the drinker has harmed is an important part of AA's program. But generally the idea of evil and wickedness is no longer held. It has given way to the concept of alcoholism as a sickness or disease.

The medical model   In this approach alcoholism is considered a disease. Physical addiction is seen as a symptom of some underlying structural or physiological disorder. The drinking is not deliberate behavior on the part of the drinker. Rather, it is due to the disease and the responsibility for the care of the alcoholic is medical. The nature of the disease called alcoholism is considered to have one or more physical bases: genetic-constitutional, biochemical, or brain dysfunction.

Is alcoholism inherited?   The search for some genetic basis for alcoholism has led to a wide range of investigations. There is some evidence that is consistent with a hereditary point of view, but these findings are not at all conclusive in that the same results can be accounted for just as well by other factors.

Research studies have shown that when compared to the general population there is a greater occurrence of alcoholism in the families of alcoholics. These studies show that there is a greater risk of alcoholism occurring in members of families in which there is at least one alcoholic member than in families with no alcoholic members. It has also been found that families with an alcoholic member also have a higher occurrence of members who have other psychopathology, namely, personality disorder and affective disorder.

Studies that have compared identical and nonidentical twins also show some support for genetic factors in alcoholism, but such data are not at all conclusive. While identical twins who have the same genetic makeup are more likely to be concordant for alcoholism (i.e., if one twin is alcoholic, the other one will be as well) than are nonidentical twins who have the genetic similarity of brothers and sisters, the concordance rate is not impressively high.

If alcoholism is inherited, it is important to know what specific factors related to alcoholism are transmitted. There is only speculation with regard to this. One thing suggested is that a characteristic inherited is an affective or mood disposition. Those born with a predisposition toward depression might turn to alcohol as a self-medication. Another view is that it is the personality disorder that is inherited. According to this approach, a general inherited antisocial approach predisposes alcoholics to drink.

Some studies have suggested that people may be born with very great differences in sensitivity to alcohol. For instance, adopted children of biological parents who are alcoholic have been found to have higher rates of alcoholism than adopted children whose biological parents are not alcoholic. Another theory suggests that a defect in the body's ability to use certain food substances causes certain people to be inclined to drink more and become alcoholic. This defect results in a dietary deficiency believed to be vitamin B complex.

Endocrine theory   The endocrine theory proposes that alcoholism is the result of a glandular disorder. The theory most widely held currently is that alcohol intake affects the adrenal glands in such a way as to cause a sharp rise in the adrenal hormone level in the blood which is experienced as a very pleasant sensation. It is followed by a sharp drop in blood level and a loss of the good feeling. More alcohol is then needed in order to get back to the initial pleasant effect.

Brain dysfunction   The theories on brain dysfunction are based on the idea that enough heavy drinking will gradually destroy brain cells. The result is that the individual's capacity for judgment and will power is weakened. It has also been found that many heavy drinkers have a history of childhood symptoms of hyperactivity and other behaviors associated with minimum brain syndrome. In general, this theory proposes that damage to the brain either from alcohol itself or brain damage due to other factors is the cause of alcoholism.

Biochemical view The biochemical theory looks at alcoholism as resulting from a disorder of appetite regulation. Certain people have a sensitivity to some of the food elements found in alcohol. These food elements cause a rapid energy and mood pickup, but they also cause a quick and sudden letdown which leads to the craving in order to prevent the uncomfortable state experienced in the letdown. This is very similar to the endocrine theory

The medical model certainly has some utility. It has been criticized by Szasz (1972) who says that calling alcoholics sick robs them of their freedom and responsibility for themselves and their acts. It also gives false hope with regards to a cure through some physical means. But it has taken away much of the moral stigma about alcoholism and it has brought alcoholism to the place where it is now considered a treatable condition.

Psychological models The psychological models of alcoholism include the psychodynamic theory, learning theories, and personality theories.

The psychodynamic theory This approach makes the assumption that drinking alcohol can and does, especially for vulnerable people, facilitate gratification of certain impulses. Without drink these impulses would not be acceptable to the individual, and they could not otherwise satisfy them. Alcohol may, by reducing the anxiety experienced due to conflicts, allow the individual to express impulses that would not be acceptable otherwise. In addition, drinking alcohol may gratify dependency needs by allowing the expression of more immature childish wishes. Further, it may as well at the same time serve as a sort of punishment for indulging those impulses. In one psychodynamic view alcoholism is seen as paralleling an infant's obtaining passive gratification by taking in by mouth in a manner similar to an infant at the breast or bottle. From this standpoint, the alcoholic is often viewed as having limited emotional development and to be functioning at a dependent, childlike level with low frustration tolerance, immaturity, and poor ability to delay gratification.

Learning theories of alcoholism These approaches to drinking view alcohol addiction as being due to the pleasant effects of alcohol that follow very soon after alcohol ingestion. Drinking becomes associated with reduced discomfort. The drinking behavior is thus strengthened by the pleasant effects which results in it happening increasingly more often when the person feels tension and discomfort. Those who do not experience much tension will not gain much benefit from alcohol, but those who suffer high anxiety will receive great relief. Such people are the ones who will develop habitual drinking patterns. While in the long run the effects of alcohol are anything but pleasant, such as hangovers and social embarrassment, these are later effects. A person learns the drinking habit because the immediate effects are pleasurable, and it is for this reason that the habit is maintained although the long-term effects are punishing.

Personality theories   While there is no agreement on whether or not there is such a thing as an alcoholic personality as such, there are a number of personality characteristics that are said to be commonly found in alcoholics. These theories describe alcoholics as being emotionally high strung, immature in relationships, having low tolerance for frustration, not being able to express anger adequately, being frustrated over unmet dependency needs, and having low self-esteem but still being grandiose in behavior. Other characteristics include being perfectionistic, being compulsive, feeling socially isolated, and having confused sexual identity.

Cultural model   This view reasons that if alcohol functions mainly to reduce anxiety, then there will be more alcoholism in cultures in which stress is more prevalent. Anthropologists report that tribes that have very marginal hunting and gathering economies do have more drunkenness than those that have better economies. Further, the drinking patterns of a given group are also related to such factors as their attitudes toward abstinence from drink, the use of alcohol in rituals connected with religious ceremonies, the social drinking pattern of the group, and how drinking for personal self-interests is regarded.

Some additional theories of alcoholism include transactional interaction which conceives of drinking as a process of playing interpersonal games in order to influence and communicate with others. The social deviate behavior theory views alcoholism as a deviation from the norm so as to fulfill the labeled role of the alcoholic.

Although most of these theories fit some aspects of the data on alcoholism, and consequently have something to recommend them, no one theory in any comprehensive way really explains alcoholism. Rather, it appears that while a given individual alcoholic may be most understandable in the terms of one theory or another, the majority of cases are understandable only in terms of combinations of factors. Certainly at this stage of knowledge of alcoholism the contribution of all areas interactively appears to be the most useful road to understanding.

Physical effects of alcohol

Alcohol basically is used or metabolized by the liver. Chronic and heavy intake of alcohol may result in both malfunction of the liver and severe destruction of the cells in the liver itself.

Hyperuricemia, the condition known as gout, is associated with an effect of alcohol that causes a decrease in uric acid extrusion. Other disorders having to do with the body's inability to use certain food substances result from changes in the liver functioning due to alcohol. One of the most frequent of these is an imbalance of blood sugar, and severe hypoglycemia (an abnormally low concentration of sugar in the blood) may result.

In addition to disturbances of liver functioning, actual destruction or changes in the liver cells can occur from chronic alcohol intake. These include the condition called *fatty liver*, with symptoms of abdominal pain, and *alcoholic hepatitis*, a condition in which there is an inflammation of the liver and destruction of liver cells. Fever, jaundice, and abdominal pain are common symptoms in this condition.

The most serious of the liver disorders associated with alcohol is *alcoholic cirrhosis*. In this condition the liver enlarges and hardens and there is clogging of the liver arteries. When the condition becomes severe, there will develop an enlargement of the abdomen. At this stage a real danger of hemorrhaging and coma is present. In the male there may be signs of development of feminine physical characteristics.

Diseases of the nervous system associated with alcoholism

Acute intoxication from alcohol can have severe effects on the central nervous system resulting in symptoms such as stupor or coma or even death.

Acute alcoholic withdrawal   It has now been shown that withdrawal symptoms can occur even when the drinker is not malnourished. In its mildest form, withdrawal reaction may be present after only a few days of steady drinking as indicated by symptoms of tremulousness and irritability. The extreme alcohol withdrawal pattern occurs in three stages of increasing severity: (1) Tremors and hallucinations reach their peak about 24 hours after the drinking has stopped. The hallucinations usually are the most obvious behavior and involve misinterpretations of the environment and hallucinations of animals and insects. When the hallucinations are auditory, they usually are of voices that are threatening, but the patients usually do not appear to be disoriented or confused. (2) Generalized convulsive seizures, often of the grand mal type, may occur between 7 and 48 hours after stopping alcohol intake. (3) Delirium with continuous tremors, agitation, nausea, diarrhea, and excessive perspiration are found between 72 and 96 hours following the cessation of alcohol intake.

Alcohol withdrawal symptoms are due to the rather sudden freeing of the central nervous system from the chemically caused depression of the system by alcohol and not the result of malnutrition.

Organic syndromes Malnutrition, particularly in the form of vitamin deficiency, is frequently found in individuals who drink heavily. Malnutrition occurs because most heavy drinkers are not interested in food and have poor eating habits when drinking. This can very seriously affect the central nervous system and can cause brain damage. Interestingly enough, the majority of alcoholic patients from higher socioeconomic levels generally are not malnourished.

Wernicke's syndrome Wernicke's syndrome is a brain disorder that results from a thiamine deficiency. It is frequently found in chronic alcoholics. The presenting symptoms develop over about the period of a week and consist of confusion, memory loss, staggering walk, and inability to focus the eyes. This condition is usually reversible by thiamine administration.

Degeneration of the cerebellum Degeneration of the cerebellum may also be related to nutritional deficiency on the basis of alcoholism. It is characterized by symptoms of staggering walk, incoordination, spasticity, tremors of the arms and legs, inability to focus the eyes, and impaired speech.

Korsakoff's psychosis Chronic organic brain syndromes that result from alcoholism also include Korsakoff's psychosis. The symptoms of this disorder are disorientation, confusion, loss of recent memory, and a tendency to fill in memory gaps with made-up stories. The patient is alert and responsive and has no other impairment of the senses. Whether the Korsakoff's psychosis is due to direct effects of alcohol or nutritional deficiency effects of alcohol is still unknown. Some of its effects are reversible by vitamin therapy. This condition almost never occurs without being associated with chronic alcohol intake.

Neurological diseases indirectly related to alcohol include *hepatic encephalopathy* which results from severe liver impairment. This disorder may include intellectual impairment and other organic brain impairment symptoms as well.

Subdural hematoma This condition is frequently found in alcoholics and is due to head injury from falling, fights, and accidents. It is a fairly common cause of death in alcoholics. Headaches, confusion, irritability followed by drowsiness, urinary incontinence, and stupor may be symptoms.

Alcohol also appears to have effects on the maturing brain of human embryos. A pregnant woman who drinks circulates the alcohol through the brain and system of the unborn. It has been reported that the offspring of alcoholic mothers fail to develop well and that infant mortality among them is high.

Sleep disturbances   Sleep disturbances are among the most frequent symptoms found among heavy drinkers. Insomnia is a common complaint and has been found in approximately one-third of alcoholics studied. This is a surprising symptom in view of the fact that alcoholism is a depressant of the central nervous system. The sleep disturbances are most often found when there are high levels of alcohol in the blood and during the withdrawal period.

Alcoholism from a psychodynamic view

From a psychodynamic point of view, alcoholism is a disorder due to psychological factors; it is not caused by physical factors. The problem behavior is the continuing intake of large amounts of alcohol. The reasons why some people do this is not always clear. Alcoholics seldom are able to give a reasonable explanation for their excessive drinking. But they do become dependent on alcohol and then are very concerned about having alcohol in sufficient amounts to produce intoxication. They are very likely to spend their time with other heavy drinkers. As they become more dependent on alcohol, the alcoholic may try to hide his or her dependency by drinking alone or sneaking drinks. This, however, is usually associated with feelings of guilt and remorse that may incline the person to drink more in order to seek relief. These feelings of guilt and remorse may be especially strong in the morning and this may become a motive to drink again to alleviate the feeling. Further drinking over a long period commonly results in anxiety and depression, and the alcoholic tries to gain relief from these symptoms through more alcohol. A vicious cycle of drinking, depression, and drinking thus may be set in motion to form the classicial syndrome. Alcoholics experience blackouts with periods of memory loss. These blackouts can cause great anxiety because the alcoholic does not know if he or she has harmed someone or has done something foolish during that period. These memory losses are such that the alcoholic has good remote and immediate memory but cannot recall what happened during the most recent 5 or 10 minutes.

The start of the drinking pattern for males tends to be in the late teens or early twenties. Definite dependency on alcohol may not be apparent until the thirties. Recent findings indicate that the development of alcoholism does not follow any clear pattern and may be quite variable. *Gamma alcoholism* is characterized by a problem of control. Once started, drinking gammas are unable to stop until poor health or lack of money force it. But once the bender is terminated, the gamma alcoholic can abstain for various lengths of time. In contrast to gamma alcoholism, the French pattern or delta alcoholism is one in which the drinker has control of how much but cannot abstain. He or she must have that given amount of alcohol everyday but has no need to exceed that amount.

The complications in all aspects of living resulting from drinking are considerable for alcoholics. Alcoholics have a high rate of marital discord and divorce, difficulty in employment, and a high rate of accidents. Approximately one-half the highway accident deaths are associated with drinking drivers and one-half of the convicted criminals are alcoholics. The medical problems resulting from heavy drinking are also considerable. Death due to depression of the breathing center or hemorrhaging may occur. Gastritis and diarrhea are common, as is gastric ulcer and liver damage. Much of the nervous system disorders are primarily due to vitamin deficiencies. This is not, however, a direct effect of alcohol. Rather, it is the result of poor diet while drinking. Wernicke's syndrome and Korsakoff psychosis are other severe conditions that are associated with withdrawal patterns. Suicide, too, is often associated with alcoholism, particularly in men over thirty-five.

The two psychiatric diagnoses most commonly associated with alcoholism are character disorders and sociopathy.

Personality measurement and prediction of alcoholism

It has often been stated that there is no personality type that is typical of alcoholics, at least prior to their alcoholism, but recent research suggests that this may not be an accurate statement. With a certain amount of consistency, alcoholics are frequently characterized by clinicians as having personality traits of emotional immaturity, social isolation, and poor personality integration. In addition, they are often described as having poor impulse control, low frustration tolerance, and feelings of unworth, guilt, and depression.

Personality test findings and attempts at predicting alcoholism

Using the Human Figures Drawing Test, a study of men in the Norwegian navy by Irgens-Jensen (1971) found a clear relationship between excessive drinking and the way human figures were drawn. Significant correlation between heavy drinking and features of the drawings were found over a number of variables. From that data the author suggests that the use of alcohol functions (1) to relieve anxiety, (2) to satisfy dependency need without damaging the male image, and (3) to facilitate fantasy about personal worth and achievement.

Studies in which alcoholics and nonalcoholics were asked to make judgments about themselves when sober and when drunk indicate that the nonalcoholics rated themselves the same in either state and that alcoholics tended to rate themselves more positively when drunk than when not.

The Minnesota Multiphasic Personality Inventory (MMPI) test has been widely used with alcoholics. Surprisingly consistent group profiles of alcoholics in treatment have been found. These are characterized by high score elevations on the psychopathic deviant and depression scales, and to a lesser extent psychasthenia, schizophrenia, and mania. These patterns suggest that neurosis, depression, sociopathy, and neurotic anxiety are common in alcoholics.

The MMPI has also been found most useful for measuring significant improvement in adjustment of alcoholics who complete treatment. The pre- and post-MMPI scores commonly show marked improvement on the depression scale. Differences between alcoholics who complete treatment programs and alcoholics who do not have been found on the psychopathic deviant (PD) scale. The PD scale seems to be the best predictor with regard to response to treatment. The higher the PD scale the poorer the response. The MMPI appears to be a sensitive instrument for measuring improvement of alcoholics during treatment and its clinical scales are useful for predicting treatment outcomes.

The absolute elevation of scales is an important part in interpreting the MMPI, but there are some quite consistent highest two-point scale findings with alcoholics as well. Common high-scale combinations found for alcoholics are as follows: PD-D or psychopathic deviant and depression scales; PD-MA or psychopathic deviant and manic scales; and PD-PT or psychopathic deviant and psychasthenic scales.

There are a number of specific MMPI scales designed to predict alcoholism. Of these the *MacAndrew scale* (1965) and the *Rosenberg scale* (1972) appear to have the most promise. One study using college students attempted to predict which students would later become alcoholics. The MacAndrew scale was able to successfully predict those who would. The MacAndrew scale pattern did not change appreciably from the time when it was given to the subjects in college to the time later when they were in treatment for alcoholism. The MacAndrew scale seems to hold promise for detecting alcohol susceptibility before the onset of overt symptoms.

There are considerable similarities in MMPI patterns between alcoholics and those who abuse other drugs. Alcoholics generally are higher on depression, while abusers of other drugs seem to have more overall personality disturbance. Narcotic addicts tend to have the PD-MA profile peaks which describe a sociopathic, emotional, and unstable personality. The more typical alcoholic profile is a D-PD-PT code described as depressive-psychopathic deviate with passive/aggressive personality features. Alcoholics seem to be more neurotic, depressed, anxious, passive, and dependent, while narcotic addicts are more antisocial, amoral, impulsive, irritable, hostile, and psychopathic.

In a longitudinal study McCord and McCord (1960) evaluated subjects initially in 1935 and did a follow-up in 1956. They report that the early personality characteristics that were later associated with those who later became alcoholics were overconfidence and a masculine facade.

In summary, there are certain pathological personality patterns as measured by several different instruments and methods that have been found to be consistently characteristic of alcoholic populations. The personality trait pattern on which these studies agree consists of depressive, neurotic-depressive, sociopathic, and anxiety features. Dependency, impulsivity, and immaturity are also frequently mentioned. However, whether such traits are factors leading to alcoholism or are only the result of it is not clear. It is also true that those same characteristics are found in other disorders not associated with alcoholism. Some MMPI alcoholism scales, particularly the MacAndrew scale, have been effective in identifying prior to addiction who would become alcoholic. A few longitudinal studies suggest the prior existence of certain personality patterns in alcoholics. But chronic drinking also results in an increase in these symptoms, particularly those concerned with depression, insecurity, and defensive behaviors.

Intellectual deficit and alcohol

While alcoholics show impairment on a number of psychological tasks, their general intellectural capacity does not appear to be greatly impaired. On standard tests of intelligence alcoholics as a group score at average to superior levels. However, impairment is noted on certain other types of tasks such as numerical ability, motor coordination, finger dexterity, etc. Poorer performances by alcoholics on perceptual organizing have been found. The block design of the Wechsler Adult Intelligence Scale also often shows a deficit performance. Spatial scanning and planning impairment have been noted on the Trail Making Test. A field dependency orientation as measured by Embedded Figures performance is characteristic, and the perceptual motor functioning on the Bender Gestalt Test is intact. Further, cognitive impairment has not been found associated with alcoholic blackouts. However, alcoholics are typically impaired on the Halstead-Reitan Categories Test. They also do poorly on the Proverb Appreciation Test.

Impairment on the Halstead-Reitan Battery as a whole has been found for alcoholics but not as severe as that found for patients with traumatic brain injury. There appears to be an increasing decline in cognitive capacity as the length of time of alcohol abuse increases. Progressive loss of the ability to maintain and shift learned concepts occurs as the duration of alcoholism increases. One theory suggests that use of alcohol over a long period leads to accelerated aging of the nervous system. However, that chronic alcohol abuse results in broad, general brain deterioration is not really supported since many of the symptoms of such disorders are noted when the individual is drinking but not observed when the individual is sober.

There is some evidence to suggest that the right half of the brain is more affected by alcohol than the left. Very consistently alcoholics show greater impairment on performance than verbal subparts of IQ tests. Typically, the test performance of alcoholics shows nonverbal and spatial relationship deficits. There is also evidence to suggest that at least some alcoholics may have suffered from hyperactivity or there may be other indications of minimal brain damage for some period before the onset of alcoholism. There is thus some evidence to suggest that the person who becomes alcoholic as an adult may have shown evidence of some degree of brain damage as a child.

Research on the reversibility of some cognitive impairments of alcoholics shows that after periods of about one year of sobriety, significant recovery does occur and improvement may continue for up to a year more. It is possible that while permanent damage may have taken place, the individual's ability to compensate for lost function by learning new ways to cope or by other brain areas taking over may account for much of the improvement.

Alcoholism and cognitive styles

Cognitive styles refer to the characteristic manner in which people express and organize their intellectual activities. One cognitive style is called *field dependence-independence*. This has to do basically with whether a person largely responds to clues and information from sources internal to himself or herself and thus is called *field independent* or responds thoroughly to the clues and information external to himself or herself, in which case the person would be considered *field dependent*.

The Rod and Frame Test has been mainly used to determine field dependence or independence. In this procedure a frame surrounding a rod can be tilted to various angles. How accurately an individual can tell whether it is the rod or the frame that is tilted is a measure of the individual's degree of field dependence or independence.

As a group, alcoholics have been consistently found to be more field dependent than other patient groups, even when hospitalization, socioeconomic, and psychopathological variables have been controlled. Further, most studies have shown that field dependence in alcoholics remains the same whether they are intoxicated or not. Also alcoholics who have stopped drinking still remain at the same field of dependence level as they were before starting to drink. Long-time drinking patterns have also been found to have no effect on field dependence. There are, however, a few recent studies in which, interestingly enough, alcoholics do show a change in field dependence toward more independence following recovery from the alcohol (Danahy and Kahn, 1981).

Generally, however, it appears that alcoholics do not show change in field dependence. Thus, the association of field dependence with alcoholism suggests that field dependence could be a predisposing or necessary characteristic for alcoholism. One hypothesis that has been raised to account for this is that perhaps field dependence represents a symptom of brain damage. Since alcoholics often are malnourished, smoke heavily, and may suffer much head damage, they are more likely to have had brain damage than are others.

While field dependence has been measured differently in different studies, there is a consistent and overwhelming amount of evidence for a high degree of field dependence for alcoholics as a group. But it is also true that a few alcoholics are field independent. The vast majority, however, fall into the dependent category. While the weight of evidence is that field dependence is characteristic of alcoholics even before they drink, it has been suggested that the dependence may be rather the result of brain damage associated with drinking. This formulation of characteristic perceptual dependency on the field is consistent with postulations of a general personality pattern of dependency in alcoholics as put forth by clinical personality theorists.

Physiological effects of alcohol

As the level of alcohol in the blood system increases, there is an arousal type of behavior response usually shown in laughter, excitement, talkativeness, and a general happy mood. As the level of blood alcohol decreases, that is when alcohol is being eliminated from the system, the usual reaction is that of feelings of tiredness, sleepiness, and general depression.

While there is a popular belief that there is some difference in the effects of alcohol as a result of the type of alcohol drunk, these differences are not great. Particular products that result from brewing called *congeners* can, however, have some slight effect on physical measures and the experience of hangover.

The concentration of alcohol in the beverage is clearly important with regard to how rapidly the alcohol is absorbed in the blood. Interestingly, a 30 percent concentration is absorbed more rapidly than either a 15 percent or 45 percent concentration. The larger the dose of alcohol, the greater the effect. Further, the effects of alcohol can be affected by eating. Slower absorption of alcohol takes place when there is food in the stomach than when there is not. Fast, rapid drinking results in greater performance deficit than sipping drinks.

When tested 15 to 20 minutes after the start of drinking most people appear excited, feel happy, and respond as if they have had a stimulant. However, their performance on tasks may be impaired. Once a peak of blood alcohol level has been reached and begins to decline, people usually become depressed, sleepy, and quiet. But their performance during the descending blood alcohol level returns almost to normal.

It has been hypothesized that certain ethnic groups have lower incidence of alcoholism because they are more sensitive to its physiological effects and thus will drink less or respond differently to alcohol. Orientals, for instance, show a greater blood flushing response to alcohol than do Caucasians. Similar responses have been reported for American Indians. But it is of note that Orientals have a very low alcoholism rate, while Indians who have a similar physical reactivity have a very high alcoholism rate. This suggests that both cultural and psychological, as well as physical factors, need to be considered.

In general, there is little consistent evidence on a distinct psychophysiological relationship to alcoholism. The physical effects of alcohol intake on nonalcoholics are about the same as are the effects on alcoholics. One of the effects found most consistently about alcohol is that of a sleep disturbance that seems to be the result of drinking. The effect of alcohol appears to be that of normalizing the sleep pattern in situations of mild drinking, but with continued drinking it leads to long-run sleep interference.

Laboratory observations of alcoholic behavior

Through the control over the drinking situations that laboratory studies can provide it is possible to test out clinical observations as well as try new procedures that would otherwise not be possible in the usual environment of the alcoholic. They have the disadvantage, however, of being artificial situations and thus the findings must be considered carefully. Laboratory studies have found, for instance, that alcoholics do take in large amounts of alcohol over long periods of drinking. But when the alcohol is available in unrestricted amounts, alcoholics do not try to drink it all up. Also, comparisons of alcoholic and nonalcoholic drinkers find that the alcoholic drinkers are more likely to choose straight than mixed drinks, to gulp their drinks rather than to sip them as the nonalcoholics do, and to drink past the stage of drunkenness more often than nonalcoholics do.

In one study which allowed choice between drink or socialization, skid row alcoholics almost always chose alcohol to other people. They often even chose to drink alone during periods of socialization.

It has been found that most people, including alcoholics, are less depressed and anxious during the time they are drinking. However, there are some alcoholics who become increasingly anxious and depressed when they do drink. This may represent two types of alcoholic: the anxiety alcoholic and the anxiety reduction alcoholic. The basis for drinking could be very different for each type.

There are other findings which indicate that people who consume beer and distilled spirits show more aggression than those who use soft drinks. However, in one study people who believed that they were drinking alcohol but were not were more aggressive than those who thought they were only drinking tonic water. In this study the ones who actually drank alcohol were no more aggressive than the ones who did not.

The widely held view that alcoholics have an increasing loss of control over drinking and an increasing desire for alcohol has not been confirmed by several of these laboratory studies. Given free access to all the alcohol they wanted, alcoholics in these studies did not utilize it. Furthermore, many chronic alcoholics are known to return to voluntary moderate and controlled drinking on their own. Thus, it appears that the involuntary loss of control theory is not well supported.

Social factors have been found to be related to drinking patterns. The drinking behavior of a drinking group's leader influences how much the members of the group will drink. If there are group decisions about drinking, the leader's opinion will also affect the pattern. Socialization seems to facilitate drinking in most alcoholics, but there are some who are inhibited by it. Studies to determine whether alcoholics will drink to reduce stress have usually used a laboratory situation with electric shock as the stressor. These studies show no support for the stress reduction model of alcoholism.

Thus, laboratory studies confirm some clinical impressions about alcoholics and refute others.

How much drinking do Americans do: Survey findings of drinking behavior in the United States

A national survey (Cahalan et al., 1969) found that 68 percent of adult Americans drink at least once a year and that 12 percent fit the category of heavy drinkers. More recent surveys suggest even more drinking currently, particularly among women and younger individuals.

The greatest proportion of heavy drinkers have characteristics of being men in their forties, being of lower socioeconomic status, living in larger cities, and being of Irish or Latin American background. Jews and Episcopalians have the highest proportion of drinkers of any religious groups; however, both groups also have extremely low rates of heavy drinking.

Those who abstain tend to be older people of less than average income from the south or rural areas. They tend to be native born and from conservative or fundamentalist Protestant denominations. It is of interest that three-quarters of those who responded to the survey indicated that they thought drinking does more harm than good.

There have been four nationwide surveys of prevalence of specific drinking problems. The categories of drinking problems usually have been as follows: (1) frequent intoxication, (2) binge drinking, (3) symptomatic drinking (Jellinek's gamma alcoholism), (4) psychological dependence, (5) problems with spouse or relatives, (6) problems with friends or neighbors, (7) job problems, (8) legal-police problems, (9) health problems, (10) financial problems, and (11) belligerence associated with drinking. Forty-three percent of the men and 21 percent of the women reported that they have had some amount of one or more of these drinking-age problems during the preceding three years.

The surveys also reveal a definite tendency for high rates of drinking problems to occur among younger men and for lower rates among older men. This is a bit of a surprise since it is the forty-plus age group which makes up the usual alcohol clinic population. It would seem from this data that a great many individuals who show the signs of serious drinking problems at an earlier age will show considerably less drinking several years later.

Socioeconomic status People of lower socioeconomic status have higher proportions of abstainers from drink than those of higher status, but those from lower status who do drink are more likely to be heavier drinkers than other persons. Also, lower socioeconomic status people have a higher proportion of drinking problems than do higher socioeconomic status people. The lower social class people also experience more difficulty from their drinking than do the higher socioeconomic group.

Religion   Most Jewish males drink some, but drinking causes trouble for only very few. Most Catholic and liberal Protestants drink and an above average proportion of them do get into difficulty over their drinking. Conservative Protestants show a high degree of abstinence.

Evidence from the survey suggests that if a person's attitude toward alcohol is very positive and if the person is in an environment that is favorable toward heavy drinking, these conditions will be very influential in increasing the probability that a young person will become a problem drinker later in life. The indications from the survey data, however, are that symptoms of a specific drinking problem are not a very accurate predictor of later drinking behavior. There will be many misidentifications of who will and who won't be later problem drinkers in attempting to utilize such symptoms as predictors.

A portrait of the chronic alcoholic can be drawn from the survey information. He or she is most likely an individual from an ethnic-cultural background that is permissive and encouraging about heavy drinking, has a history of childhood neglect or rejection, has come to put an evaluation on alcohol as the way of dealing with problems, and has personality characteristics of poor self-regard, and of little tolerence for delaying gratification which are traits consistent with using alcohol to escape. The survey shows that positive attitudes toward heavy drinking and drunkenness are found very frequently among young urban men.

Furthermore, it appears that such a favorable attitude toward alcohol is the best single predictor of drinking problems. From this it would seem that changing attitudes and values toward drinking are what are needed for prevention. It is very likely that such a basic, favorable attitude toward alcohol is the crucial reason why half of those who contact alcohol programs never follow through with treatment.

In terms of prevention, the survey points out the fact that only a large-scale social change carried out by a grass-roots person-to-person evangelizing could change social norms sufficiently to where moderate drinking could be socially controlled. It might be useful to study ethnic cultural groups such as Jews and Chinese, most of whom drink but few of whom develop into problem drinkers, in order to find which factors might be fruitful for developing preventive programs.

Culture as related to alcoholism

What is considered to be alcoholism, as is the case with abnormal behavior, varies from culture to culture. Horton (1943) hypothesized that drinking in any society is related to the level of anxiety in that society. He looked at primitive groups in which economic and cultur-

taking place the patient should be watched for the early symptoms of the DTs, for the DTs can be prevented. The basic symptoms and signs of the DTs may be noted as early as from 24 to 36 hours following the cessation of drinking.

The symptoms of the DTs are any or all of the withdrawal symptoms and confusion, hallucination, extreme agitation, and fever.

The basic medical treatment for alcohol withdrawal involves injection of chlordiazepoxide (Librium U.S.) for the anxiety and agitation symptoms and vitamins (thiamine particularly to ward off Wernicke's syndrome and Korsakoff's psychosis). The use of diphenylhydantoin sodium (Dilantin U.S.) is used to deter convulsions which are a real risk in alcohol withdrawal. Keeping up proper fluid level to maintain hydration and electrolyte balance is essential.

Pharmacologically, alcohol detoxification is viewed as replacing the alcohol with a comparable sedative drug which in turn can be smoothly withdrawn. A wide number of tranquilizers and sedatives have been tested for this purpose and it has been found that Librium is the most effective and avoids side effects as well. Librium and several other drugs have also been demonstrated to be effective when the patient is in active DTs (Cole and Ryback, 1976).

Outpatient detoxification has been successful in a great many cases. It is also clear that many alcoholics manage to detoxify themselves without medical help. The hangover dealt with by a Bloody Mary, which provides the addition of a small amount of alcohol for gradual withdrawal and some nutrition, may serve that purpose. If there has been prolonged heavy drinking, it is risky.

Successful outpatient detoxification requires voluntary desire by the patient and involvement of other significant people such as the drinker's family or friends. It is also necessary that the patient live within a reasonable driving time to the place where drying out is to take place. In the usual outpatient detoxification program the patient receives medication, is immediately involved in peer group activities, and family or friends are also quickly brought into the rehabilitation program. The requirement that the alcoholic come back to the clinic every 12 to 24 hours for further medication is a big help in developing a supportive relationship for the alcoholic. Librium is probably the medication of choice for outpatient detoxification.

Conditions that need to be met for effective outpatient detoxification are that the patient must agree to return the next day, that only one day's supply of medication is given at a time, and that a moderate withdrawal reaction is anticipated.

Following detoxification many alcoholics experience depression and anxiety similar to that which impelled them to drink in the first place in order to avoid these painful feelings. For that reason, antianxiety and antidepressant drugs are sometimes used during postdetoxification treatment. However, studies of these drugs, as well as of Lithium, have compared them to placebos. They do not have any dramatic effects on the depression and/or anxiety of postdetoxified alcoholics.

Alcoholics Anonymous

It was during the period when there was little or no help and interest from professional sources that Alcoholics Anonymous was started. It got its start from Dr. Bob and Bill W. (following AA's practice of not identifying members by their last names). AA membership has grown to an estimated almost one million members currently in 195 countries throughout the world. At least 14,000 AA groups are active in the United States. In 1970 there were 427 AA groups in Australia.

Alcoholics Anonymous is a self-help organization of alcoholics helping other alcoholics. The following is a paraphrase of the description of AA which is often read at the beginning of regular AA meetings: AA is a fellowship of men and women who share their experiences, strengths, and hope in order to solve their common problem and to help others recover from alcoholism. The only requirement is a desire to stop drinking. AA is self-supporting, but there are no dues or fees. Members contribute, but the amount of contributions has an upper limit. It is not affiliated with any religious group or political or business organization. It avoids controversy and does not endorse or oppose causes. The primary purpose is for members to stay sober and to help other alcoholics achieve sobriety. There is no provision to punish members or to exclude them from AA.

The basic AA principles for recovery and continued abstinence from alcohol are stated in the 12 steps of AA. They are in essence as follows:

1. To admit powerlessness over alcohol and that one's life has become unmanageable.

2. To come to believe that a power greater than oneself can restore the alcoholic to sanity.

3. To make a decision to turn one's will and one's life over to the care of God as God is understood by the individual.

4. To make a searching and fearless moral inventory of oneself.

5. To admit to God, to oneself, and to another human being the exact nature of one's wrongs.

6. To be entirely ready to have God remove all the defects of one's character.

7. To humbly ask God to remove one's shortcomings.

8. To make a list of all persons one has harmed and to become willing to make amends to all.

9. To make direct amends to such people whenever possible, except when to do so would injure them or others.

10. To continue to make personal inventory and when one is wrong to promptly admit it.

11. To seek through prayer and meditation to improve one's conscious contact with God as one understands God, praying only for knowledge of God's will and the power to carry that out.

12. Having had a spiritual awakening as a result of these steps, try to carry the message to other alcoholics and to practice these principles in all of one's affairs.

The philosophy underlying these principles is aimed at two main characteristics of the drinking alcoholics: (1) their defiance and independence and (2) their defensive and exaggerated sense of their abilities. Through admitting their powerlessness and through acknowledging a power greater than themselves, these two factors are deflated, which then allows them to turn to a superior power and to others for help. This occurs only after there has been some intense personal soul searching and the making of restitutions for damage they have done. A very important part of AA is that the program is carried out in the spirit of a close, warm, supporting group that provides a sense of belongingness and worth to the alcoholics for taking these steps.

Alcoholics Anonymous meetings are of two types: open and closed. Anyone is welcome at the open meetings where various members will often tell the history of their drinking, how it affected them, and where they stand now. The closed meetings, for members only, are for more intimate and intense discussions of these problems. However, there is much AA activity that occurs outside the meetings in the form of informal social contacts. Members often visit or phone each other and a sponsor makes himself or herself available anytime and anywhere to help a new member.

Alcoholics Anonymous reported some figures on the effectiveness of its methods for obtaining its primary goal, that of sobriety. The sobriety figures reported by AA are that 35 percent of those in AA who are sober for less than a year will not drink and will remain in AA the following year. Of the 65 percent remaining, most will still drink and may or may not stay in AA. However, most of them do stay in AA and try again. Only from 5 percent to 10 percent of this total leave AA. Of those in AA who stay sober for from one to five years, 79 percent will not drink and will remain in AA. The remaining 21 percent will either become inactive in AA but stay sober, or will leave AA and resume drinking, or will drink and start AA over again. Of those sober more than five years, 91 percent will not drink and will remain in AA. It is clear that the longer the period of sobriety, the better are the chances for remaining sober.

These figures indicate that to stay sober for a full year is most difficult, but if that is accomplished, the chances of staying sober for the next few years are much improved. Even so, approximately one-third will begin drinking again. However, for those who can remain sober in AA for five years, the risk of falling back into drinking again is very low.

It should be pointed out, however, that since AA is a voluntary program, it undoubtedly means that there is considerable selectivity in who goes there for help in the first place. The 12 steps are demanding and require strong motivation to be able to complete them. The effectiveness of AA may not be different from that of other programs that also demand a strong motivation to quit. But AA has demonstrated that it can succeed when working with people who are really motivated to quit drinking.

Alcoholics Anonymous has also developed two important related organizations, *Al-Anon* and *Alateen*, which have been developed to work with family members of alcoholics. The purpose of these group programs is to help the other family members to accept and realistically deal with the alcoholic member's behavior. Alateen is for the children and the younger members of a family in which one or both of the parents are alcoholic. Al-Anon is basically for the spouse or adult members of the family of the alcoholic.

Alcoholics Anonymous has made a very positive contribution, not only in terms of its effectiveness for those who have the motivation to become involved in an AA type of program, but perhaps more importantly, for its pioneering work in proving that alcoholics can be helped. Alcoholics Anonymous stepped in when no one else was interested or would risk trying. AA's concept of the affected person being the primary source of help for another affected person has been shown to be an effective treatment strategy. The AA model has been used widely in other areas.

In recent years there has been a major shift in viewpoint and today alcoholism is recognized as a major social and health problem. Considerable money is now going into treatment and research. While AA remains a very important method for treating alcoholics, there are now available other approaches that can be considered and used.

Anti-alcohol conditioning drugs

Another widely used approach to treatment of alcoholism involves the application of certain drugs that when taken in the correct amount will interact with the alcohol in the body in such a way as to cause extremely distressing effects. The main drug of this kind is *Antabuse*, chemically known as disulfiram. When the amount of Antabuse in the blood is at the appropriate level, the ingestion of alcohol will result in symptoms of flushing, sweating, palpitations, dyspnea, hyperventilation, hypertension, nausea, and vomiting. The person will experience extreme discomfort.

Antabuse has been in use for alcoholism treatment for more than 30 years. It seems to be effective with a certain limited number of patients, but there is reason to believe that the taking of Antabuse sometimes has effect because it is more a test of desire to stop drinking than it is an effect of the drug itself. Patients who are successful with Antabuse tend to be older, socially stable, very motivated to stop drinking, better able to form dependent relationships, less depressed, and less likely to have blackouts or sociopathic traits than are other alcoholics. Many consider that Antabuse is not a cure but that it can be very useful in providing support to aid in avoiding impulsive drinking for those who have real motivation to stop. It is a method to help an individual maintain control over drinking. It is recommended that it not be given to organically confused, psychotic, severely depressed, or suicidal persons.

Other drugs used in alcohol treatment

In treating withdrawal symptoms Librium has been shown to be a safe and effective drug that can reduce or eliminate the DTs. Promazine has been found to increase the occurrence of the DTs and is associated with a higher death rate than any other treatment method. Thus, it is contraindicated. The antianxiety and antidepressant drugs have not been shown to have any very clear effectiveness in treating detoxified alcoholics in the community. Antabuse, as has been noted, is useful for certain individuals who are motivated because it can help them maintain self-control. In general, creating avoidance of alcohol by using nausea-causing or paralyzing drugs has not been shown to be effective. These drugs may serve only to be indicators of motivation. LSD, which has been used as an adjunct to psychotherapy with alcoholics, has not generally been shown to have any effect.

Psychotherapy methods and procedures with alcoholics

Traditional psychotherapy methods that are used with neurotic patients, such as psychoanalysis and dynamically oriented insight therapies, generally have not been effective when used with alcoholics. Similarly, poor results have been found with the client-centered approaches as well. This probably is related to the fact that such therapies are based on substantial motivation on the part of the patient to change and that much of the responsibility for the therapy process itself falls on the patient.

However, most alcoholics enter into therapy as passive participants who are there because of external pressure. They may have no real motivation to quit drinking and are only seeking medical help in order to dry out. Most alcoholics approach treatment with the expectation that the therapist has the major responsibility to treat them. Alcoholics may deny having any serious personal problems or may not see any significant relationship between problems and their drinking. Alcoholics typically do not want to face their more basic reasons for drinking. They tend to deny problems and do not even understand that it is possible to have another lifestyle. For many, alcoholism is the only basic career they have ever had. Alcoholism is at least the only career with which they feel they are successful and at ease. This means that therapies must involve considerable intervention and action by the therapist in order to reach such alcoholics. In group therapies the danger is that these kinds of alcoholics may support each other's passivity.

One psychotherapeutic approach which has been reported to work with alcoholics combines individual and group therapy ongoing at the same time (Fehr, 1976). The therapy is done in a group situation. The seating arrangements are such that at one end of the circle of chairs for the group there is a chair for the therapist and an empty one for a given patient. In this method the therapist does an intensive diagnostic interview of each of the alcoholic patients in front of the group in order to identify the problems and the patient's style and manner of dealing with them. Some group involvement in this assessment is allowed, but it is considered as basically individual work with the patient. Each of the patients has a turn to be in the working chair. Approximately 20 minutes is the maximum time during any one session for any given patient. The therapy first works mainly as individual therapy. The goal is to establish a broad behavioral diagnosis. As the group members become acquainted with each other's situation and problems, their input to the situation is gradually brought in. The therapist must be very active in such groups and must frequently step in. But the therapist should be careful not to do the therapeutic work for the individual. Rather, the therapist should encourage the patient and group members to do it on their own.

This approach is an adaptation of traditional methods and seems to have considerable promise for working effectively with passive and poorly motivated alcoholics.

A wide variety of group therapies have been used as part of alcoholism programs. These have been carried out from a number of different theoretical vantage points. Most frequently they have been drawn from the standpoint of Transactional Analysis, Synanon Games, and Gestalt therapy. In more than a few ways, such groups develop a group atmosphere similar to that provided by Alcoholics Anonymous. It may well be that a similar kind of principle provides the effect. But such therapy groups usually are only part of more comprehensive programs and the evaluation of their effectiveness is not clear.

Behavioral approaches to alcoholism treatment

Earlier behavioral focus for treating alcoholism was on the use of aversive procedures such as electric shocks and noxious chemicals. These generally have not been effective. What results that have been found appear most likely at this point to be due to more general treatment factors than to the aversion procedures as such.

The current social learning model views alcohol abuse as a socially learned behavior pattern. The pattern is maintained by a variety of rewarding or reinforcing effects of a psychological, sociological, or physiological nature. These reinforcers include such things as reduction in anxiety, increased social attention or approval, being able to be more outgoing and spontaneous socially, and the avoidance of physiological withdrawal symptoms, all of which can cause drinking behavior to continue.

There are a variety of behavioral methods. The behavioral approach based on operant procedures would require first a detailed assessment of the specific preceding and consequent events related to the excessive alcohol intake. Then a baseline level of drinking behavior before treatment is found. For example, by recording time, place, and circumstances of each drink over a specified period and by following this procedure with the use of social learning techniques, new social skills would be taught that could provide alternate satisfactions to drinking. Then the person's natural environment would be rearranged so that the consequences for drinking are not rewarded but those for sobriety are. Finally, evaluation of the effects of these measures would be carried out by comparing the initial baseline amount of drinking with the amount of drinking after the treatment.

The first part of the behavioral treatment is an assessment of the relationship between the drinking and the factors associated with it. This assessment is made by looking at what precedes the drinking and at what the immediate consequences are for the individual. The baseline data are very important since from that the therapy plan can be worked out and an evaluation of the therapy can be made. The baseline information comes from the patient's own report, from reports of observations by people close to the alcoholic, and by direct observations by the therapist. Such reports must be as detailed as possible. For example, they should include as much of the following information as possible: (1) the time and date of each drink, (2) the particular type of drink; (3) the percent of alcohol in it; (4) the number of sips per drink, (5) how much of the drink was consumed, and (6) the place and circumstances in which the drinking was done.

There are many other behavioral assessment measures that can be helpful. These include procedures for measuring how much work an alcoholic will do in order to obtain a drink, observing the amount the alcoholic will drink when alcohol is easily available, and determining what the alcoholic's attitude is toward alcohol.

Research has now fairly well established that there is a significant relationship between satisfactory social, emotional, and occupational functioning and success in alcoholic treatment regardless of the treatment method used. Predictively then, it is important to know how well an alcoholic is functioning in his or her overall life situation. It is also important to determine the conditions that are maintaining the alcoholism for the given individual. The treatment can then be directed toward developing new conditions and new responses. If, for example, an evaluation indicates that what is needed is to alleviate anxiety, or improve self-esteem, or develop better social relationships, then such means to change the impetus for drinking can be developed by using these indicators to find new responses.

Finding appropriate alternatives to alcohol is the next step after the behavioral assessment. Alcoholics are often found to have poor skills in such areas as socializing, self-management, relaxation, and in vocational and recreational functioning. Behavioral treatment programs thus usually focus on training the alcoholic in these skills. Assertiveness training is a procedure that has been used very widely. It is discussed in more detail in Chapter 10. It is a method whereby the person is trained to effectively satisfy his or her needs and wants without being overly aggressive or harmful to others on the one hand, while being able to comfortably assert himself or herself appropriately on the other. For example, alcoholics might be taught how to refuse drinks when in a situation in which there is much social pressure to drink. Learning how to refuse firmly but in a manner that doesn't offend and developing increased self-esteem and self-confidence are included. In addition, learning the skills needed to deal and cope with marital problems and other social relationships and learning improved occupational and recreational skills are all important aspects of the behavioral approach to finding alternatives to drinking.

The behavioral approach also works to change the consequences or results of the behavior of the alcoholic. For instance, removing the great attention the alcoholic often receives for drunkenness, even though it is negative attention, takes away a reinforcement for drinking. In its place the alcoholic is given a maximum reward for abstaining or moderate drinking to provide an alternate behavior. These methods require the assistance and cooperation of friends and relatives. Token economy and signed contract methods also may be helpful in this regard.

Finally, a behavioral evaluation of the patient's behavior change from his or her initial baseline is made in order to determine the effectiveness of the treatment.

Other therapeutic approaches

In addition to the treatment approaches for alcoholism reviewed here in some detail, there have been a great many other psychotherapeutic approaches and programs applied to the treatment of alcoholics. Many of the encounter-humanistic group treatment methods, including Transactional Analysis, Synanon Games, and Gestalt therapy, have been used extensively with alcoholics.

Treatment programs should not lose sight of the fact that alcoholics often live in a family relationship, at least initially, until their drinking results in a broken family. Today alcoholism is viewed as not just the problem of the individual alcoholic but also the problem of all the family members. Consequently, family therapy is another frequently used treatment method for alcoholics. The general approach and techniques and family therapy have been discussed earlier.

Conclusions

From what has been reviewed here about alcoholism it should be clear that it is a very complicated problem, and it follows that there is no one method of cure and there are no simple, clear, direct, and immediate solutions. Alcoholism often involves many physical problems; at times it can be a medical emergency. Alcoholism can also lead to permanent destruction of body organs and parts of the brain. There may be hereditary aspects to the susceptibility to alcoholism, but very strong psychological and social factors are also involved.

Consequently, treatment is never simple. In most cases, it should involve a number of interrelated and cooperating approaches, the particular balance of which probably needs to be worked out for each given case.

Clearly, a comprehensive community approach to treating alcoholism is needed. Such an approach should include emergency services for the emotional crises of the alcoholic and the alcoholic's family, as well as for the medical crises that may be involved in acute intoxication, particularly including detoxifcation. This suggests that inpatient hospital services for alcoholics are in certain instances necessary. Once the acute crisis is past, many alcoholics need a transitional program such as a halfway house, nursing home, live-in group home, or partial hospitalization. These various living arrangements should include programs that have not only shelter and medical attention but also psychological counseling and rehabilitation programs. Outpatient facilities for alcoholics who can be treated on an outpatient basis are a necessary part of a total program. These services should include psychological support, individual and group treatment, medication, vocational assistance, and socialization.

A community outreach approach is especially needed for alcoholism programs since there is so much reluctance on the part of alcoholics and their families to become involved in existing programs. Outreach programs operate through workers who can identify drinking problem situations and then advise and encourage the identified alcoholics and their families to come into treatment. This way those with drinking problems can be reached earlier and effective treatment can start before more serious consequences occur.

After-care and evaluation of the program's effectiveness are also important and must be part of a comprehensive program.

In terms of what factors predict improvement with regard to drinking, recent studies have indicated that the psychosocial level of functioning before treatment is the best. Further, the younger the individual, the shorter the period of heavy drinking, and the better the employment and education level, the greater the improvement (Emrick, 1975).

Prevention is the ultimate aim of such comprehensive programs. Although the demands for service work with the affected alcoholics are great and it may be difficult to convince funding agencies of the importance of time for education and training, preventive work needs to be done. Prevention should be given high priority, and there should be special emphasis on youth, both in the home and in school.

summary

1   Defining alcoholism is difficult because there is no one typical pattern of drinking. The out-of-control, increased tolerance type is probably best known but it represents only some cases. A definition that covers most conditions is: intermittent or continued use of alcohol with dependency or harm in mental, physical, or social spheres.

2   Theories on the causes of alcoholism include the older traditional moral model which blames the alcoholic as a willful abuser for his or her own pleasure; the medical model which views alcoholism as a physically based illness; psychological models which stress psychodynamics or learning; and a social-cultural model.

3   The physical effects of alcoholism include a variety of medical conditions such as alcoholic cirrhosis of the liver, withdrawal effects including the DTs, and neurological brain disorders such as Korsakoff's psychosis.

4   Despite the general rejection of the idea of an alcoholic personality, certain consistent personality test patterns have emerged, especially on the MMPI, that are characterized by peak elevations on the psychopathic deviant and depression scales and by psychoasthenia, schizophrenia and mania.

5   Alcoholics show certain specific cognitive impairments but general intellectual abilities are intact. Alcoholics have been found to be consistently perceptually field dependent.

6   Although there are some ethnic differences in the response to alcohol, the physiological effects of alcohol are not different for alcoholics and nonalcoholics. Orientals and Indians have a strong flushing response to alcohol, but Orientals generally have a low rate of alcoholism while Indians have a high rate.

7   Survey data found most heavy drinkers to be men in their forties, to be lower socioeconomic individuals in large urban areas, and to be of Irish or Latin-American descent. Permissive attitudes toward drinking and a permissive drinking environment favor the development of alcoholism.

8   The first effective treatment approach for alcoholism was Alcoholics Anonymous. AA's treatment approach is based on the 12 steps in which alcoholics must admit to their powerlessness with regard to alcohol and to a power greater than themselves. Alcoholics Anonymous documents a reasonable record of success.

9   Aversive conditioning methods with alcoholics, such as the use of Antabuse, seem to work only when the person is strongly motivated to quit, and hence they may be basically measures of motivation.

10   Withdrawal or detoxifcation is frequently necessary and can be done on an outpatient basis, but it may require hospitalization. Use of chlordiazepoxide, vitamins, and anticonvulsive medications often are required.

11   The standard psychotherapy methods do not generally work with alcoholics, but specialized methods such as using active, directive therapists have been successful. The behavioral method emphasizes developing substitute skills and responses for drinking such as assertive training and socialization skill learning.

12   There is no one effective treatment method. Motivated patients who stay in treatment six months or longer do well regardless of the method used. A comprehensive community approach, one that includes prevention, is recommended.

Special intervention methods briefly

There are a great number of psychological, social, and medical intervention procedures available today and only a few of them have been given in detail in earlier chapters. Most of these additional intervention methods can be used in and of themselves as fairly complete treatments for certain types of problem. But these methods may also be used as supplementary techniques in support of other more general treatment procedures. For instance, in marriage counseling which might have as its goal to basically improve the relationship and communication between a couple, it might well be helpful to include assertive training for one partner who might be having difficulty letting his or her needs be known. Certain sex therapy techniques for that couple might prove helpful in the overall treatment as well. Even psychopharmacological drugs might be indicated for reducing anxiety.

This chapter will consider briefly six additional treatment intervention modalities so that mental health workers can be aware of these methods and their potential uses. These will include the role of the patient advocate, how the social welfare system works, behavior therapies, assertive training, sex therapy, and therapeutic drugs for emotional disorders.

The role of the patient advocate

Mental health problems involve people's entire lives. Very often the stress and difficulties faced by an emotionally disturbed person are partially or largely due to the stresses of the persons's economic, family, or social situation. But it is also true that individuals with severe emotional problems may do things which help create difficulty in their social relationships and their economic and family situations. The treatment then usually must involve not only dealing with the individual's psychological reactions but also helping the person to cope and come to grips with these other circumstances. This suggests that the mental health practitioner may at times find it necessary to become involved in helping the patient find and appropriately use the welfare and social service resources available. The mental health practitioner will find it useful not only to know what social benefits and programs are available but also, even more importantly, how these benefit systems work. Furthermore, the practitioner should know what is necessary in order for the patient to receive benefits.

Traditionally the role of mental health personnel has usually been limited to evaluation and treatment of an individual's emotional disturbance. When the patient had problems involving a need for welfare or social service benefits, the patient was referred to the agencies that deal with such matters. Thus, social and welfare problems were kept separate from mental health treatment.

There has been an increasing awareness that the social and financial problems that cause the patient to seek these social welfare benefits are very much a part of the emotional problem and should not be separated from it. Thus, helping with such matters should be considered an equally important part of the patient's overall treatment.

The most frequently occurring situation is when people who are emotionally disturbed require a great deal of direction, support, and help in order to obtain the needed social welfare benefits. In recent years there seems to have been an increase in the complexity of the available benefits, with ever increasingly complicated regulations and involved forms to be filled out. The task of applying may present an almost overwhelmingly difficult situation for the person who is emotionally distraught and does not understand the procedures of such agencies or for a person who has had little education or has poor communication skills.

In some mental health programs certain personnel have become *patient advocates*. They help the patients find the services or benefits they need. They work closely with the patients to help them through the maze of bureaucratic requirements. In order to function as patient advocates, they must have a broad extension of the usual mental health skills and knowledge.

There is some controversy over whether or not patient advocacy is a proper role for mental health personnel. In our view, it is a necessary service and sometimes it is a crucial service from the standpoint of the patient's treatment. Mental health workers can very appropriately perform this role, but whoever does it, it is often crucially important if the patient is to be best served. The patient advocate role can be seen as an additional treatment skill for mental health workers, but it should be only one of the many skills of the mental health worker. If it were to become the sole function, the role would be too limited, and it would deal with only a small segment of a patient's total life situation. Achieving social welfare benefits alone for the patient may be part of mental health treatment, but it is not mental health treatment all by itself. The social benefits advocacy role should thus be only part of a more total mental health worker's range of intervention skills.

So far we have talked about the need for social benefits for patients who are first identified as having emotional disturbances. Should mental health services assume the advocacy role for people seeking only help with social benefit problems? Such cases should be evaluated carefully. Many people in need of social welfare benefits are under great situational stress and frustration. It may well be that their emotional disturbance is an important factor and a main reason why they are in the situation that requires them to seek such benefits. Helping such people obtain social welfare benefits provides the mental health worker with a means of developing a broader relationship with them, which can become the basis for dealing with their mental health problems as well. Otherwise, they may remain too inaccessible to be helped with their emotional problems. In such situations, a social welfare benefit advocate role as part of mental health treatment seems indicated.

For those cases evaluated as not having a significant emotional component but just involving a need for benefits, a referral to the appropriate agency would probably best serve those involved and allow mental health workers time to deal with cases that are more appropriate to their overall skills.

An example of how this can work is the case of George who came to a mental health clinic seeking assistance in obtaining welfare benefits. The reason he needed them was found to be closely related to his mental health problems. George was a 33-year-old man who had been drinking heavily for several months. He had drifted from town to town, sometimes obtaining odd jobs in order to obtain money for alcohol, but more often he joined with drinking groups and obtained alcohol from them. He had been staying at a public park drinking with a group and sleeping under the bushes. George came to the clinic seeking money so that he could return to his home. He had no income whatsoever and no place of shelter and he had not eaten in two or three days. Furthermore, he had been unable to obtain much to drink in the last few days and was beginning to become shaky and tense and appeared to be verging on delirium tremens (DTs). In a semidrunken state, George insisted that he only wanted welfare assistance and had no other problems. A mental health evaluation pointed to not only an alcoholism problem but also to a severe depression lasting for several years and starting when his wife took his three children and left him. She refused all his efforts to have her return and soon was living with another man. That is when George's drinking began to greatly increase and he soon lost his job. From that point he began his aimless wandering from place to place and existed in a drunken state most of the time.

It was decided that George would be a good case for a mental health advocate to work with. George was helped with gaining some of the needed social benefits, thereby enabling the mental health worker to develop a relationship with him. Through the relationship the mental health worker hoped that he could influence George to face and deal with the problems in his life, including his current alcoholism.

Initially, George was told that his mental health worker advocate would assist him in gaining the benefits but first George would have to shower and shave and put on some clean clothes, as well as sober up before he could hope to convince the welfare agency of his need. George agreed to this. Overnight shelter at an alcohol rehabilitation center was found for George and his mental health worker advocate accompanied him there.

In the morning, with some assistance from the program staff at the center, George was adequately cleaned up, and the mental health worker advocate found out what documents were needed in order for George to receive benefits. The advocate accompanied George to the proper office. George did not have the necessary papers, but he was eligible for some emergency funds. Before that could be completed, however, George became quite ill from alcohol withdrawal and was taken by the advocate back to the alcohol rehabilitation center where he was treated for several weeks. The mental health advocate visited him every day and developed a good counseling relationship with him. George was successfully withdrawn from alcohol. He continued to work with the mental health worker around his feelings about what had happened with his wife several years ago and about ways of controlling his drinking.

George was finally able to complete the necessary papers in order to receive welfare benefits which included money for emergency travel back to his home area. When George left, almost a month after the original contact, he had been without drink for almost all of that period.

He was in very improved health and nutritional status, and he was determined to return to his former home area where his friends and his type of work were available. There has been no further word from him since he left.

Whether or not George received sufficient help to have overcome his drinking problem and to have learned how to deal with some of the problem situations of his life is unknown. But the point of this case example is more concerned with how the roles of the patient advocate and mental health worker fit together in a particular case. Had it not been for the mental health worker's interest and knowledge that helped George to receive welfare benefits, he very likely would not have become engaged in treatment or have been willing to go into the alcoholic rehabilitation center. He needed the social benefits and in this case that was a central means of engaging him in a broader treatment process.

How the social welfare system works

Benefit systems and social service programs almost always operate under fixed and sometimes very rigidly fixed rules and regulations. Since most often these are government programs, the agencies are required by law to hold to certain regulations. Beyond that, however, the agencies may put their own interpretations on some of the rules, or sometimes individuals working for those programs interpret the rules in a fairly personal way. Mental health personnel must know the rules and requirements for the various benefit programs so that they can help their patients receive assistance. In addition, they must know how these rules are being interpreted so that they can present the right kind of information in order to receive benefits.

If the patient advocate feels that the rules and regulations have not been interpreted accurately by the agency, the patient advocate can help the patient to appeal the case. Here a basic knowledge of the system (what it provides and what its rules are) is very necessary. Of equal importance is a knowledge of how the system actually works. Mental health practitioners should become very familiar with the available benefits and services and with the procedures and personnel of each program. Mental health workers who have personally experienced dealing with programs to obtain benefits for themselves and their families are often especially aware of the many difficulties people face in trying to gain benefits for which they are eligible.

Almost all agencies require that an applicant for their services or benefits fill out an application form. The forms ask for basic information about the applicant, for example, name, address, birth date, marital status, family size, income, and so forth. These forms may be very long and frequently they are very difficult for people who are upset or who have poor reading and language skills to understand. The agencies may also require proof of authenticity of the individual's statements.

As an example, in order to be eligible for health care at one county's expense, patients must bring as much of the following information about themselves as possible:

1. *Identification:* Driver's license or other ID with picture; birth or baptismal certificate; social security card, medicare card; immigration card or naturalization papers; welfare or public assistance card; marriage license or divorce papers.

2. *Income Over the Last Thirty Days:* Verification of total income and sources of income through (a) paycheck stubs, (b) employer statements showing wages, (c) check-cashing verification form, (d) letters from persons providing free rooms and meals, (e) self-employment records, (f) any other receipts of income.

3. *Resources and Assets:* (a) Health or life insurance policies, (b) bank account records, (c) titles to property, (d) certificates of stocks and bonds, (e) trust funds.

4. *Military Service Records*

5. *Medical Bills and Expenses:* A list of all expenses for medical reasons; statements and receipts.

Obviously, these are a very complicated and demanding series of requirements in order to prove eligibility for a government supported service. For many poor, uneducated people or for persons under great emotional stress, these requirements can be overwhelming. In fact, many people eligible for such services become totally discouraged by these bureaucratic procedures. Some give up and do not try to obtain the help they really need.

It can take a considerable amount of time to fill out the forms in order to get assistance. Also, considerable effort may be needed in order to obtain all the verification necessary. Knowledge about how a particular assistance agency works can help greatly. For instance, if the patient advocate knows that it may take the better part of a day to fill out all the necessary forms, the patient advocate can advise the patient to bring lunch or perhaps to arrange for a baby-sitter for an extended period. Once the forms and information are gathered, then the individual applying for benefits may have to wait in line until his or her turn to have the forms processed. This too could be a lengthy, time-consuming procedure. Furthermore, the patient should be prepared to answer challenges or questions about certain items of information. If the patient does not know how to answer, the patient may be sent back to get additional material, thus, necessitating delay and waiting for another appointment to be processed.

Personal contact with the people of the agency from which benefits are sought can be very helpful in arranging for appointments, in obtaining information on what is needed, and in gaining cooperation. To the extent it is possible, the patient advocate should spend some time getting to know the agency and the people who run it.

Each benefit system is different. The examples above only represent a few of the complications that advocates should be prepared to help their patients with.

Types of services and benefits

The number of services available to people of limited or destitute circumstances vary considerably from place to place. While many of these are governmental programs, frequently private charitable organizations offer considerable services as well.

As an example, in one particular area some of the major services provided are administered through the state government. These include the following:

General Assistance Program. Provides minimal money for food and shelter to adults who have no other means of income.

Aid to Dependent Children. Provides financial support for children whose families do not have enough money to care for them.

Aid to Families of Dependent Children. Provides funds for families in which there are children.

Emergency Relief Fund. Provides funds for stranded, destitute individuals. It is mostly concerned with providing them with minimal funds to return to their home communities.

Adoption Services (under *Family and Children's Social Services*). Arrange for the adoption of children to families which can take care of them.

Adult Protective Services. Deal with such things as family violence and mistreatment of adults within the home.

Child Protective Services. Deal with protecting children from neglect, malnourishment, beatings, and sexual assaults.

Day-Care Programs. Provide care for children whose parents are working or who cannot otherwise take care of them.

Foster Home Evaluation and Licensing. Provides alternate homes for children who cannot be taken care of or who cannot get along in their own homes.

Social Services. Provide a variety of home visits and evaluations. Under the social services are included *Food Stamp Eligibility,* a program that provides basic foods at a lower-than-retail cost for individuals of income who qualify.

Job Services. Help individuals find work.

Mental Retardation Services. Provide various levels of training and institutionalization for mentally retarded individuals.

Unemployment Insurance. Provides financial benefits over certain periods of time for individuals who have worked but are currently out of work.

Veterans Affairs. Coordinates special benefits available to veterans.

Vocational Rehabilitation. Evaluates and trains individuals and often provides treatment and therapy in order to prepare people to be able to hold jobs.

The *Social Security program* of the federal government has benefits for *disabled workers* and *their families.* This general program is for those who have previously worked under Social Security and are currently unable to continue. Evaluations of the disability are made, and those eligible are paid sums according to their disability. The *Old Age Survivors Benefits* of Social Security provide retirement income for individuals at certain age levels and *Survivors Benefits* if the individual dies prior to being eligible for the retirement benefits.

Health services

Every community has various health services of which the patient advocate should be aware, particularly those for which poor people would be eligible. These include hospitals and clinics specially designated for taking care of people who have little or no income. Especially noted should be the special health services clinics, such as prenatal clinics, children's clinics, venereal disease clinics, and alcoholism detoxification clinics.

The mental health facilities and the mental health services and programs they provide and the clientele with which they work should also be well known by the mental health worker advocate. If clinics are set up to serve only specific geographical areas, this should be known by the mental health worker. Specialized services in mental health provided in *child guidance clinics, drug* and *alcohol programs, halfway houses,* various *counseling centers,* and *emergency walk-in* mental health services should all be considered.

Mental health workers should be aware of and be able to provide information to their patients on the availability of *emergency food* and *emergency shelter.*

Areas of community supports and benefits

In addition to the more formal government welfare benefits, in almost all communities there are a number of facilities and agencies which may be available to assist people in need. Those working in the mental health system, and particularly those who are working in an advocacy capacity, should know about these resources and agencies and know where they are and how they operate.

Law enforcement includes, among others, the *police* and *sheriff* who may be of assistance in many ways aside from their usual known functions. For instance, they can help locate lost persons. Probation departments for both adults and juveniles are important contacts. Cooperating with probation officials may be very helpful in finding jobs or living arrangements for patients. Schools often have special resource police who can in some cases be of assistance.

Legal aid is a vital service that provides legal assistance, usually free of charge, to people in need. In addition, there are a number of different types of legal officers, such as the *public defender,* the district attorney, and judges. Courts are often specialized to deal with juvenile, domestic, or criminal matters. Thus, a knowledge of the legal system is useful and often necessary.

Some communities have *emergency telephone services,* which include information about *hospitals* and *emergency medical services* and provide telephone numbers for the *fire* and *police departments, child protection agencies, rape crisis centers,* and *women's centers,* and for the *Red Cross, Alcoholics Anonymous,* and so forth. *Transportation services* also may be provided in emergencies by ambulances, the fire or police departments, or by various centers which service people.

Mental health workers should become familiar with the emergency rooms of available hospitals, with the various police and fire rescue squads, and with available clinics. Hours of operation, what each specializes in, and the location of each must also be learned. Mental health workers must also know about places offering immediate walk-in counseling and crisis treatment.

The various *shelter care* facilities for indigent persons should be known. These might include the *Salvation Army,* the *YMCA* and *YWCA,* and *St. Vincent de Paul,* which provide a place to eat and/or sleep. Mental health workers should be familiar with the location of low-cost shelter and food accommodations.

In summary, the kinds and types of facilities vary from community to community. The mental health worker should become acquainted with the various facilities in his or her area. It is very useful to compile a complete list of such agencies and include information on where they are located, their hours of operation, and what services they provide. The mental health worker should also visit and make personal contact with all these agencies and develop good, friendly working relationships with the personnel. Such efforts are very much in the best interests of a mental health worker's patients and they make the accomplishment of the job more possible and satisfying.

Behavior therapies

Behavior therapies are widely used methods of treatment for behavior disorders. They are based on the principles of learning that have been developed from laboratory experiments with animals. Behavior therapies generally proceed on the assumption that behavior difficulties are due essentially to either faulty past learning for a given situation or to not having learned certain skills needed for coping with a problem situation. Behavior therapies consider the disorder to be only those precise observable behaviors the individual shows in certain current problem situations. Through applying the principles of learning, behavior therapists work to change the immediate behavior responses. The method is not usually concerned with past history or with any aspects that are not directly related to the actual behaviors involved in the difficulty.

For example, a child considered to be hyperactive and unmanageable by a teacher would be viewed by a behavior therapist as responding to the situation with a series of actions that are maladaptive. These actions would be designated, such as running around the classroom, talking at the wrong time, and so forth. Once the exact behaviors targeted for change have been identified, behavior therapy proceeds to use learning principles in an effort to change them.

Classical conditioning

There are three main approaches to changing behavior by learning principles: classical conditioning, operant conditioning, and modeling. In *classical* (or *respondent*) *conditioning*, which seems to be fairly automatic, the kind of response that ordinarily is brought on by one type of occurrence can be brought on by a very different one. For instance, a sudden loud noise will, in most people, usually produce a fright reaction in which there is a tensing of the body and heart pounding. If just before a sudden loud noise a cat were to walk in front of a person, especially if this were to happen several times, then the sight of the cat alone could produce the fear and physical reaction. This is how behavior therapists consider a phobia or an irrational fear is caused. In the case of the example above, it is an irrational fear of cats.

A conditioned fear can spread, that is, it can generalize from the original cat to all cats, or even to all furry animals. A conditioned fear can also be lost by weakening the connections. This could happen if the cat is seen enough times when a loud, frightening noise doesn't happen.

An effective way to deal with such an animal phobia would be to countercondition it (Wolpe, 1969). This involves changing the association of the cat with the fearful noise to pairing the cat with something pleasant and relaxing. In the procedure called *desensitization*, a series of situations are worked out to consider from least to most what circumstances cause upset in connection with a cat. For instance, looking at a picture of a cat in a book might cause little upset. This would be done along with relaxation exercises until the person becomes very comfortable while looking at pictures of cats. Then the next least frightening situation with a cat would be enacted along with relaxation, progressing until the person with the cat phobia can, let's say, be relaxed while holding a cat and petting it.

Operant conditioning

Operant conditioning is based on the kind of result, positive or negative, a given behavior brings. If a given action is followed by a positive result, that action has an increased likelihood of being repeated. If the result is negative, the action is less likely to be repeated. In this method, the way to get rid of an unwanted behavior is to make sure that it is not followed by a positive result. For instance, if a child, as the result of a temper tantrum, receives a great deal of attention, even if the attention is negative, then the child is more likely to have tantrums frequently. But if the tantrums are regularly ignored and the nontantrum behavior is given attention, then the tantrums have a high likelihood of decreasing or stopping and the more positively received nontantrum behavior has a high probability of increasing.

Similarly, the way to have a wanted behavior occur more often is to be sure that when the wanted behavior occurs it is followed by a positive outcome. For instance, children who can only make sounds but do not talk have learned to say words by being directly rewarded with small pieces of candy for sounds that are anywhere close or similar to the sound of the word and then by being rewarded for sounds that are closer and closer approximations of the sound until the sound of the desired word is given. With this procedure it has been possible to "shape" certain behaviors and have them occur regularly when initially these behaviors were not even present. But in order to learn a response by this method, the response or something approaching it must be given in order to be rewarded (Blackham and Silberman, 1975).

Modeling

Modeling is based on the principle that people learn by observing the actions of others. The more similar the one who models the behavior is to the learner, and the more respect the learner has for the model, the greater the likelihood that the model's behavior will be learned. A boy, for instance, may learn how to throw a basketball by watching other boys or from watching television (Bandura, 1971).

The various learning methods when used for treatment have proved to be very effective for a variety of problems. Their best success has been in training young children and in working with severely handicapped and retarded individuals.

Assertive training

Assertive training is one of the learning-based techniques that is used when a problem is related to inhibitions or fearfulness about doing or saying things which are reasonable and well within the rights of the person to say or to do. Some of the reasoning here is that fear and inhibitions prevent or interfere with a person's ability to satisfy his or her needs. As a result, the individual experiences frustration and does not function very effectively within the family or in society.

Assertive training is also used with individuals who express their needs and desires in socially unacceptable ways. Such behavior may cause them many difficulties in dealing with their families or with society in general. An example would be a person who frequently has temper outbursts or someone who is so aggressive and demanding in sexual behavior that he or she offends and drives the partner away. This person must learn to express his or her needs realistically in socially acceptable ways, not in a crudely aggressive manner.

The nonassertive person is often an individual who because of a strong sense of guilt or anxiety or a deficiency in social skills has difficulty in expressing his or her feelings, whether they are loving or angry ones.

Some of the false assumptions that nonassertive individuals often follow and that need to be corrected are: (1) The assumption of modesty—the idea that it is good to be modest no matter what. However, it should be realized that by giving selective information about one's accomplishments and strengths, one can help strengthen relationships instead of weaken them. (2) The assumption that a good friend, spouse, relative, neighbor, or anyone who if he or she really cared should know one's needs and feelings and give without the need of having to be told about them. To really care is to do for the other person without being asked. If one has to ask for something it isn't worth anything. One must learn that others can't read his or her mind and must learn how to let others know his or her wants. (3) The misconception that showing or experiencing anxiety is a sign of weakness. Men particularly are often afraid to show fear or to take a chance in a situation in which they are afraid because it might expose them as seemingly weak. Bravery is doing something in the face of fear, not being fearless. (4) The assumption that in order to maintain a relationship or friendship one must always give in to others' requests. Relationships require give and take, and others respect those who can stand up for their own needs.

An aggressive person is one who may get most of his or her needs met, but often at the expense of the dignity or self-respect of another person. Such a person may express anger on slight provocation, put others down by calling them names, dominate conversations, attack, and criticize. Of course, the person ends up with very poor relationships with others. It should be clear that assertive training is not training to be aggressive.

Assertive training works to reduce anxiety that occurs in interpersonal situations so that the person is not afraid to assert himself or herself and is comfortable in developing the skills required to satisfy his or her needs. Assertive training begins with helping the person to understand the reasonableness of asserting and gratifying his or her own needs and interests and doing it in a socially acceptable way.

Assertive training then generally goes on to determine what the problem areas are that the individual wishes to work on and change. Along with this is a determination of the amount of anxiety and concern with each situation. Then goals on what things are going to be changed are set. Once these goals are established, invoking the various procedures of practice statements, role playing, and homework assignments are carried out to make the change.

In initially assessing an individual's assertiveness, the Assertiveness Inventory of Alberti and Emmons (1974) is sometimes a very useful tool.

Wolpe (1969) uses five questions to get some idea of the assertive posture of a patient. The questions may not be appropriate for certain cultural groups, in which case other more suitable questions should be devised. The areas covered by Wolpe's questions are:

1. If after buying something in a store you find that your change is a dollar short, what do you do?

2. After returning home from a store you find that something you have bought is slightly damaged. What do you do?

3. When someone goes ahead of you in a line, for example, at the movies or at a sports event, what do you do?

4. When you are in a store, and the clerk waits on someone who came in after you, what do you do?

5. What do you do when eating out and the food is not the way you ordered it?

The therapist first finds out where the patient's anxiety and fears about being assertive are most bothersome. Then the therapy proceeds gradually, working up from the place where the patient is least frightened and inhibited to levels closer and closer to the most uncomfortable situations, in a manner similar to desensitization procedures.

Patients are taught to talk freely, to express felt emotions spontaneously, and to show their feelings in their facial expressions. When a patient doesn't agree with something within reason, the patient is taught not to pretend that he or she does. Instead, the patient needs to learn to contradict the situation in a reasonable manner. Frequently training people to use the word "I," to be able to accept praise, and to give self-praise when it is appropriate are some general exercises that are useful.

For example, training clients to make assertive statements that are appropriate in various situations is also useful. A suggested list of assertive statements for certain situations, based on Wolpe's list, follows:

1. Would you call me back? I can't speak now.

2. Would you please stop talking during the movie?

3. This is a line; please go to the end of it.

4. You have kept me waiting for 40 minutes.

5. Your behavior disgusts me.

6. I can't stand your nagging.

7. I'm sorry, but it won't be possible.

8. I think that is no concern of yours.

9. I insist that you come to work on time.

10. Pardon me, I was here first.

11. I enjoy talking to you, but please be quiet while I'm reading.

Other assertive statements of a more positive nature are as follows:

1. Your dress is beautiful.

2. You look lovely.

3. What a nice smile you have.

4. I love you.

5. That was really a good job.

An important caution in doing assertive training is to be sure not to start someone on an assertive course which is likely to result in punishment. In other words, it is important to be practical in choosing assertive behaviors for practice. Situations in which results are most likely to be positive are the ones in which assertiveness will be learned.

Another technique that is used in assertive training is "one-upsmanship." This sometimes calls for special information about the other person's weakness. With that knowledge certain kinds of statements can often put the other person at a disadvantage. A widely used example to put somebody on the defensive is to say, "Is there something wrong with you today? You don't seem to be quite your usual self."

One of the best methods for developing assertive behavior is to *role play* the situation with the patient. If, for instance, assertiveness is to be developed for dealing with a clerk in a store, the patient might first take the role of himself or herself at the store and the therapist the role of the clerk. Thus, the therapist can see how the patient responds and might then suggest more effective responses to the clerk. Then the therapist and the patient switch roles. This procedure is continued until the patient becomes practiced, experienced, and at ease when being assertive in a given situation. Role playing can be used to develop comfortable assertiveness for increasingly sensitive situations.

Assertive training works through teaching anxiety reduction and providing skill training. A person who is assertive can establish close interpersonal relationships and still protect himself or herself from being taken advantage of by others. He or she can make decisions and free choices in life without experiencing undue anxiety and guilt and can do so without violating the rights and dignity of other people.

Some techniques for practice which have been useful in assertive training are:

1. *Eye Contact.* This is first practiced at a distance. Then still maintaining contact with the other person, the patient gradually moves nearer to the other person.

2. *Self-Praise.* The patient is asked to think of at least four very positive things about himself or herself and to acknowledge his or her strengths and positive things he or she has to offer.

3. *Practice in Introducing Oneself.* The patient practices being realistic while avoiding anxiety and undue humility.

4. *Practice Conversations.* The patient makes a special effort to strike up conversations with strangers or with people whom the patient would like to know better.

5. *For Defensive Assertion: Practice in Turning Down Requests.* The patient practices turning down a sales person, refusing when asked to give donations, or saying no to requests for personal or private information. Other things in this area include learning to stop other people who are verbally directing criticism at the patient and learning how to deal with the anger of others when it is directed at the patient.

6. *Practice in Giving and Accepting Compliments.* In more friendly and intimate relationships the patient often needs practice in giving and accepting compliments.

7. *Practice in Saying No to Friends Who Want to Borrow Something.* The patient learns to deal with a friend who wants to borrow something the patient needs or with a friend who is known for not returning the things he or she borrows.

Sex therapy

In recent years much progress has been made in the treatment of sexual inadequacy (Masters & Johnson, 1970). You will recall from Chapter 5 that sexual inadequacy in the male refers to impotence and to premature ejaculation. In the female, sexual inadequacy involves the general lack of sexual arousal, lack of or very infrequent orgasmic response, and vaginismus, which is a constriction of the vagina so that intercourse is not possible.

These conditions can cause severe difficulties in an individual's marriage and love relationships. They clearly affect how an individual regards himself or herself and can result in a great deal of anguish and misery. Sexual difficulties may further result in constriction of the individual's ability to function effectively and to fulfill his or her potential.

Until recently treatment of these disorders tended to stress early attitudes, guilts, and conflicts with regard to sexuality that were formed in childhood. The approach was lengthy psychotherapy to resolve these conflicts.

The newer treatment approaches emphasize current situational factors in the actual present sexual situation rather than the past history.

While in many cases the factors of earlier experiences and attitudes are important causes, nonetheless, many cases can be treated by simply considering the current circumstances. There are, however, some cases in which both past history and here-and-now factors need to be dealt with. But there are many cases in which the past influences do not appear to be important and working with the immediate situation is all that is needed. Two of the here-and-now factors are discussed below.

1. Either because of ignorance or through avoidance not doing things which are effectively stimulating and exciting to both partners. This may simply be due to a lack of knowledge about sexuality or perhaps to too much guilt or inhibition to explore and experiment. Younger women in particular need more stimulation and sensitivity for arousal than do young men. Neither may be aware that the clitoris of the woman is the focus for her erotic pleasure and orgasm. Men over 50 may not know that in order to function sexually they may now require intense stimulation from their partner, but rather expect instantaneous arousal from very little stimulation as is usual for males of younger years.

If the situation is one of sexual ignorance, the main here-and-now factor is the need to learn about the many aspects of sexuality and how they develop over the life span. Just being given permission by the therapist to seek out what sexual things give them pleasure reduces guilt, and this permission may be all that is needed. But it may also be necessary to change such false beliefs such as the necessity of mutual orgasms or that a certain size penis is needed to satisfy a woman.

Guilt and anxiety about sexuality, even when the person is not aware of it, will lead the person to avoid experiencing sexual pleasure. One result may be a tendency to stay away from sexually exciting partners or effective forms of stimulation. If such a person does have sex, he or she will tend to go about it in a very mechanical, ungiving way. The person discourages the partner from stimulating and exciting him or her and wants to be done with it quickly.

2. Another set of problems has to do with not being able to meet the demands of the sexual situation. Concerns about being unable to perform the sexual act adequately is the greatest factor in male impotency. The loss of the erection probably happens to every male at some time. Males who panic and experience it as a deep personal inadequacy or who are afraid that the erection will never return are laboring under a great deal of pressure and have grave concern about their performance in future sexual attempts. It is the anxiety about being able to perform that must be worked out in these situations.

A similar situation occurs when there is a lack of sexual response to a partner's demand for sex. The male often feels the importance of meeting the sexual demands of his partner, and being unable to perform can be particularly devastating. While a woman cannot on demand produce instant sexual arousal, she can comply on demand whereas the male cannot. When the major factor of a dysfunction is pressure to perform, then providing relaxed, nondemanding sexual situations is usually the way to deal with this problem.

Too great a need to please and satisfy the sexual partner can also have a negative effect on the sexual enjoyment of both. If the man becomes so concerned with holding back his orgasm that he becomes anxious, the whole experience and performance may be impaired.

Women are often very anxious about being rejected or not liked by the sexual partner. Some may feel that they must have a quick orgasm in order not to disappoint the partner. Some women worry that their bodies are not exciting enough, or they fear rejection if they were to ask the partner to do what would please them most.

Failure to communicate

Failure to communicate is not a cause of sexual dysfunction, but it does contribute to the problem and may increase it. For example, one partner may hesitate to ask for stimulation in the way that gives him or her the best pleasure because of fear of being rejected or considered perverse by the other partner. Such a person will continue to be sexually frustrated and often will be resentful toward the partner. When each partner is able to let the other partner know what is liked and isn't liked and what is wanted and what isn't wanted, then many of the conditions that lead to sexual dissatisfaction will not occur.

The nature of the relationship between the couple usually will have considerable effect on the quality of the sexual interaction. For instance, if the partners are too competitive with each other, or if they find each other physically or psychologically unattractive, they will be unlikely to find sex with each other meaningful or enjoyable. Other relationship factors include such things as lack of trust between the partners, power and control conflicts, and struggles that may result from regarding the partner more as a parent or child than a lover. Disappointment in one's partner because he or she has not come up to one's expectations is another source of relationship difficulty. Some couples actually overtly defeat sexual involvement. Starting quarrels or bringing up other serious problems are ways to upset the partner so that the partner loses interest and can't function sexually. Some other ways to turn a sexual partner off include choosing a time which is inconvenient for the partner or making oneself repulsive by becoming unattractively fat, smoking cigars, and not being clean. Frustrating the sexual wishes of the partner is another way to sabotage sexuality. An example would be a man who is stimulated by sucking the woman's breasts. If his partner claims to be too ticklish and doesn't allow him to do it, he can be very frustrated in the situation. Another example would be one in which one partner is most aroused in the mornings but the other insists that sex occur only at night.

General treatment procedure

Masters and Johnson (1970) have developed sex therapy procedures which are based on their research and which have been widely used. These methods do require that the therapist have extensive training and experience. In the Masters and Johnson method the therapy is limited to a two-week period and there is one male and one female therapist working with each couple. The treatment is carried out every day, including Sundays, and only couples are accepted. However, if a patient does not have a partner, a partner is found for the patient. After thorough discussion with the partners about the difficulty and the treatment goals, the next step begins with instructing the couple not to have sexual intercourse, but instead to carry out what is termed *sensate focus* exercises. In the sensate focus exercises each partner takes a turn at gently stimulating the body of the other partner, who communicates what areas and what kinds of stimulation are most pleasurable. Sexual activity of this kind involves no demand for intercourse and orgasm. It is intended to be just simple, relaxed finding out about pleasurable things in oneself and in one's partner. It is considered to be an important first step in the treatment of sexual difficulty.

The couple usually reports an increase in sexual pleasure and arousal from the sensate focus exercises. In the next step the couple is told how to carry out the specific methods for correcting the particular dysfunction.

Treatment of male dysfunctions

Treatment of male impotency or erectile insufficiency is based on the presumption that it is fear or anxiety that is essentially interfering with the man's erection. Treatment proceeds first by having the patient abstain from having orgasms for a period so as to build up the individual's sexual drive. Along with this it is important to maximize conditions in which there is a freedom from anxiety about performing and from fear of failure. Such conditions are provided by nondemand pleasuring, permission to be sexually selfish, and allowing the patient to proceed at his own pace. When the erection is regained, intercourse should proceed at a comfortably slow pace, at first with the man on his back and the partner on top of him. For the first few engagements the couple separate before ejaculation, but after that things should continue more normally. It should be noted that maintaining or initiating the erection may often require a great deal of extra stimulation on the part of the woman.

In the case of premature ejaculation, Seaman's squeeze method has been used and is very effective. This method involves having the male either through intercourse or stimulation reach the point where he feels ejaculation is about to occur. Right at this stage the stimulation is stopped. The head of the penis is then squeezed, or it sometimes is effective to just wait until the intense arousal feeling has decreased. Then the stimulation is started again. This is repeated three or four times and then the ejaculation is allowed to happen. This method is usually best carried out using the intercourse position of the female on top straddling the male because the stimulation of the male is much less this way than when he is in the male top position. Control of ejaculation develops rapidly in most cases using this method, but it does depend a good deal on the cooperation of the partner.

Female dysfunctions

The three major types of sexual dysfunctions in women include the general sexual arousal dysfunction which has in the past been called frigidity. This refers to the inability of a woman to experience much if any pleasure or arousal from sexual stimulation. Such a woman appears to not experience sexual feelings. In addition, she may not have the physiological arousal (lubrication) either. Usually such women are completely inorgastic, but this is not necessarily always so.

Another major dysfunction of the female is that of infrequent or absent orgasm. This by far is the most frequent sexual complaint of women. Generally, these women are, except for the absence of orgasm, sexually responsive, experience erotic arousal, and have the physiological arousal pattern.

Vaginismus is a very rare female sexual difficulty. In this dysfunction the vaginal opening involuntarily closes tightly whenever entry is tried. Of course, sexual intercourse is then not possible.

Treatment of female dysfunctions

General sexual arousal dysfunction For general sexual dysfunction (frigidity), the first step is to help the woman to understand her feelings, fears, and guilt with regard to sexuality and to help her to become more comfortable about her sexuality.

Sensate focus exercises are the first sexual activities in the treatment. These start with first an absence of sexual intercourse for several days, and then the only sexual activity is limited to gently touching and caressing each partner's body. Under these relaxed conditions the woman can focus on her body's sensations and find the areas that are sensitive and pleasurable. Once she begins to experience some arousal from the sensate focus procedure, some more direct but light teasing genital caressing is added to the exercise.

When there has been some positive arousal response to sensate focus, intercourse following appropriate arousal is the next step. This needs to be done, however, in a very easy, slow, and nondemanding way, and further, in a manner so that the woman can control the situation. The woman on top position is useful in this procedure because the man can stimulate the woman's genital area during intercourse which will increase her erotic pleasure. The results that have been obtained from this method have generally been favorable.

Orgastic dysfunction   This is the most common dysfunction in women. The Masters and Johnson studies show that most women do not regularly have an orgasm during intercourse. In order to be orgastic, they require other kinds of stimulation of the clitoris. There is then a wide range of orgastic response in women. Not having orgasm during intercourse is considered within the range of normal variation for women provided that orgasm can be achieved by other methods.

The treatment for inorgastic women starts with helping them to understand their sexual inhibitions, fears, and guilt. It has been frequently found that the difficulty is simply that they have never been stimulated enough in the sensitive areas to produce an orgasm.

The sexual procedure with an inorgastic woman begins with allowing her to or teaching her how to masturbate. This usually involves overcoming a great deal of guilt. It is important that the therapist give the patient permission to do it. When masturbation by hand through instruction and practice is not successful in bringing on an orgasm, then the electric vibrator is used. This can provide a much more intense stimulation. When the woman has learned how to have an orgasm, has learned to be relaxed and comfortable about it, and can allow herself to enjoy the pleasure of it, then the emphasis is changed to a heterosexual one. After regular intercourse in which the male has had an orgasm, the male in a nonpressured, nonurgent way then proceeds to bring the woman to orgasm by use of his hand or with the vibrator. After this is achieved, the next step involves intercourse using the female on top position so that the male can stimulate the woman's clitoris by hand to bring on orgasm during intercourse.

Vaginismus Vaginismus (involuntary constriction of the vaginal muscles that prevents entry) is very rare and it seems to be a learned, automatic response. In most cases, it is the result of a great deal of fear and guilt about sexuality. These psychological factors must be dealt with first; then the treatment itself is relatively simple and usually successful. It proceeds by gentle insertion into the vagina of tubes of graded diameters. The first tube is wire thin. When the patient is able to easily tolerate that size, then the next larger tube is introduced. Larger and larger tubes are used until one the size of an erect penis can be accepted without difficulty.

The results of the sex therapy methods described here have generally been positive. It should be noted that the above discussion presents only a general outline of the procedures and methods. Adequate sex therapy cannot be done successfully without a great deal of training and practice before one works with patients in this area.

Therapeutic drugs for emotional disorders

Many emotional and behavioral disorders can benefit from treatment with medicines and drugs which are currently available. It is only within the last 20 years or so that such medicines have been available and there seems to be more and more such medicines being developed. The increase is both in the number of medicines and in the range of conditions for which they may be of use.

It should be pointed out that these medicines by and large treat only the symptoms of the disorder. They do not seem to work to eliminate the basic causes. That is probably not too crucial in situations in which there is only a temporary emotional reaction. Under those circumstances, the drug can help the person over the crisis, and then the medicines are no longer necessary. However, many conditions are much more long lasting. Then the following question arises: Is it better to keep a patient permanently on a drug to relieve the symptoms, or to use the drug only as a temporary measure, or not to use the drug at all? In place of drugs the alternative would be to work with the person to help the person to eliminate the psychological causes of the problem or to help the person develop better coping skills for dealing with it. In order to make such important decisions, the mental health worker must make a very careful assessment of the patient and the patient's situation.

Generally, we take the point of view that drugs can be very helpful in some or even in many cases with which a mental health worker must deal. However, these drugs are not helpful in every case and should not be used routinely. In most cases, they should be viewed as a temporary help to be phased out quickly as the patient develops other ways of coping with the situations or problems.

There has been a great deal of criticism, and rightly so, that the drugs for emotional and behavior disorders are greatly overused, particularly when the emotional disturbance is a minor one. Anxiety and depression are, after all, very normal emotions experienced in some degree by everyone, and probably very often. People must learn to tolerate and cope with these common emotions. These feelings do have a positive value. They function as very useful signals to a person, telling the person that something is wrong and alerting the person to the need to develop some means for dealing with them. Dependence on pills for a sense of well-being may well destroy an individual's ability to deal effectively with current and future problems.

Mental health workers need to be aware of the symptoms and be-haviors for which drugs can be of assistance. Often the mental health worker is the individual closest to the patient, and, therefore, the mental health worker can assess whether or not symptoms which might re-spond well to drugs are present and can assess the effects of the med-icine once it has been started. The mental health worker is also in a position to observe whether the drugs are having the desired effect, are having too much of an effect, or are causing difficulties. Such infor-mation guides the physician who prescribes the drugs so that he or she can determine which medicine is effective and can determine the proper dosage.

These therapeutic drugs are prescribed by a physician. When a mental health worker is the primary therapist for a patient, the mental health worker should be able to recognize the behaviors and symptoms that may be helped by these drugs. The mental health worker should discuss them with the physician and should also keep in close contact with the physician about the effects of the drug.

There are drugs now available for the treatment of anxiety, insomnia, depression, mania, schizophrenia, seizures and convulsions, alcohol-ism, and hyperactivity in children. Each of these areas is discussed briefly below and some of the main characteristics of drug treatment for each of these areas are summarized in Table 10-1 at the end of the chapter.

Drugs for difficulty with sleeping and anxiety

Drugs for sleep and anxiety problems should be used when these problems are frequent and intense. Then the use of antianxiety or sleep-inducing drugs should be temporary. Anxiety and trouble sleeping are, as was noted, fairly common conditions and in most cases should not require treatment by the use of drugs.

When anxiety or insomnia (difficulty sleeping) are symptoms of other more serious disorders, then these conditions may need to be treated by other methods. Sleep disturbance, for instance, is a common major symptom of depression, which may often be better treated with anti-depressant drugs or other procedures. It also should be noted that the amount of sleep needed differs from person to person. Four or five hours may be enough for some individuals, while others may require eight or ten. Particularly as people grow older they often need less sleep and that should be considered normal, not insomnia.

The drugs used most widely and considered the best for relatively simple anxiety and insomnia are those composed of benzodiazenpines because they are relatively effective and have fewer complications than other drugs. *Valium* is a widely used drug of this type, as is *Librium*. The barbiturate drugs such as *Chlorohydrate, Seconal,* and *Doriden* are less widely used and have more serious complications. The barbiturates can be particularly dangerous in that they are addicting and an overdose can cause death. Barbiturates are particularly dangerous when taken with alcohol. Antihistamine drugs which are useful for allergies also cause drowsiness and have been used for anxiety and insomnia.

Mood-regulating drugs

The mood-regulating drugs are used for depression and for mania. They are very helpful in situations of severe and profound mood difficulties.

For depression, the tricyclic antidepressive drugs are considered the most effective drug treatment. These are sold under trade names such as *Tofranil, Aventyl,* and *Elavil*. It should be noted that these drugs are slow to take effect and a level in the system must be built up. It may take several weeks to reach an effective level. Both patient and therapist should be aware of the fact that it may take a while before the antidepressant drugs are likely to be effective.

There is another antidepressant drug called M.A.O. (monoamineoxidase) inhibitors. They tend to be generally less effective than the tricyclics and have many more side effects and complications. However, in some cases they do work better. As with the other drugs, the antidepressants, both tricyclic and M.A.O. inhibitors, have side effects which can be serious. The M.A.O. inhibitors are particular prone to complications.

The basic drug for mania or elevated, excited mood is lithium carbonate. It is sold under the trade names of *Eskalith* and *Lithane*. Lithium is effective in controlling manic behavior and preventing the repeated cycles of manic episodes. Lithium, however, requires two or three weeks to have effect and often other drugs must be used until the lithium effects can be noted.

Lithium must be medically watched very closely because an overdose can be very serious. Frequent testing of the concentration in the blood is required when a patient is on lithium.

Antipsychotic drugs

There are now a number of antipsychotic drugs available. Most of them are basically phenothiazines, but several others are now in wide use as well. These drugs often have effected very rapid improvement in acute cases of schizophrenia, with chronic cases sometimes requiring three weeks or more. *Chlorpromazine* is one of the best known of these drugs. It can bring about quieting of the patient, and it can reduce delusions, thought disorder, and hallucinations. *Thorazine, Mellaril, Trilafon, Stelazine, Haldol,* and *Moban* are some of the better known trade names.

There is now a long-acting form of antipsychotic drug which can be injected and will stay active and effective over several weeks. It is very useful for those who do not for whatever reason take medication as directed. It is known as *Prolixin Decanoate*. Since there are side effects with this antipsychotic drug, patients on it must be checked regularly.

Drugs for convulsive disorders

Seizures and convulsions due to organic brain damage can often be effectively controlled and even eliminated by the use of anticonvulsive medication. *Dilantin* is the best known trade name of these drugs. In addition to controlling seizures, these anticonvulsive drugs may also be of use for symptoms of hyperactivity, impulsiveness, and difficulty in attending when such behaviors are the result of certain kinds of brain damage.

Antihyperactivity drugs for children

Interestingly enough, it has been found that certain drugs which are energizers or mood elevators for adults may have the opposite effect on hyperactive, distractable, and impulsive children. These are the *amphetamines* (or pep pill drugs) and *Ritalin*. They require careful regulation but can in some cases be very effective with hyperactive children. However, it has been found that the caffeine in coffee and tea, which is also a stimulant drug, in many cases can have the same effect as Ritalin or the prescribed amphetamine drugs. It is thus probably useful first to try a cup of coffee or tea as a stimulant to see if the problem can be improved by this simple ordinary means before moving to the use of a prescription drug.

A general caution needs to be made about all the drugs mentioned here. In almost all cases, these drugs interact with other drugs and sometimes with certain foods as well. The effect of these interactions is often to increase, sometimes to a very great extent, the effect of a drug an individual is taking. Thus, it can be very dangerous to mix drugs, and medical guidance is needed if this is to be done. Drinking alcohol while taking these drugs can be particularly dangerous and sometimes fatal because the mix can so increase the effect of each drug that it becomes a lethal overdose.

A summary of the main classes of psychotherapeutic drugs and their characteristics are given in Table 10-1.

Table 10-1 Drugs Helpful in Treatment of Mental Health Problems

Type of Drug	Generic Name	Some Common Trade Names in U.S.	Indications—Target Problems	Therapeutic Effects	Some Common Side Effects	Cautions
Hypnotics (Sleep-inducing)	Barbiturates	Nembutal Seconal Doriden Chloralhydrate	Anxiety Insomnia	Induce sleep Drowsiness	Hangover Dizziness Ataxia Incoordination	Physically addicting Withdrawal symptoms Overdose—lethal
Antianxiety	Antihistamines	Atarax Vistaril	Anxiety Insomnia	Drowsiness Induce sleep	Hangover Ataxia Dry mouth Urinary retention	
	Benzodiazepines	Librium Valium	Anxiety	Anxiety Tension	Drowsiness Dizziness Ataxia	
	Meprobamate	Tranxene Miltown	Anxiety	Anxiety Tension	Drowsiness Dizziness Ataxia	Overdose—lethal
Mood Regulators Antidepressants	Tricycle	Elavil Tofranil	Severe prolonged depression	Decreases depression	Dry mouth Hypotension Drowsiness Weight gain Urinary retention	Requires several weeks for effect
	MAO Inhibitors	Nardil Marslid Marlan	Severe prolonged depression	Decreases depression	Hypotention Restlessness Insomnia Nausea Dizziness Constipation Loss of appetite	Requires several weeks for effect Interacts with many drugs and foods—severe reactions

Type of Drug	Generic Name	Some Common Trade Names in U.S.	Indications— Target Problems	Therapeutic Effects	Some Common Side Effects	Cautions
Antimanic	Lithium carbonate	Eskalith Lithane	Mania	Decreases mania Prevents recurrence of cycle	Thirst Fine tremor Diarrhea Weight gain Confusion Nausea and fatigue	Requires several weeks for effect Requires frequent check of blood levels Overdose toxic
Antipsychotic	Phenothiazines and others	Thorozine Trilafon Stelazine Mellaril Navane Holdol	Schizophrenia	Decreases psychotic symptoms	Drowsiness Parkinsonism Dry mouth Hypotension	May require several weeks for effect
Anticonvulsive		Dilantin Tagretal Zarontin	Epilepsy Convulsions Organic hyperactivity	Controls convulsions		
Antialcohol	Disulfiram	Antabuse	Countercondition pleasant effects of alcohol ingestion	Cause severe nausea when alcohol is ingested		Requires good health Reactions can be quite serious
Antihyperactivity (in children)	Caffeine Amphetamine	Ritalin Coffee Tea Dexedrine	Hyperactivity Distractability Impulsiveness in children only	Calming effect Improves ability to attend and be less active	Loss of appetite	Abuse potential of amphetamines high in adults

1 Several additional intervention methods that may often be useful for the mental health worker are briefly described. These include the role of the patient advocate and making use of the social welfare system, behavior therapies, assertive training, sex therapy, and psychopharmacological (drug) treatment.

2 Social and economic problems cannot be separated from emotional ones. Patients often need assistance in obtaining benefits and services from social welfare agencies. The mental health workers can appropriately and meaningfully act as the patient's advocate in this regard. Knowing how the agencies of the social welfare system work is important.

3 Behavior therapies are based on principles of learning and assume that behavior difficulties are due to faulty learning. Desensitization is an effective procedure for reducing fears and phobias, and operant conditioning is an effective method for strengthening positive behaviors and weakening undesired ones.

4 Assertive training is a method of helping a person to either overcome fears and inhibitions about saying or doing what is reasonable to satisfy his or her needs or to learn to avoid offensively aggressive behavior by learning to be reasonably assertive.

5 Treatment for sexual dysfunctions emphasizes the current situation and deals with factors of guilt and anxiety and concerns about adequacy, along with specific sexual exercises such as sensate focus and the squeeze technique for premature ejaculation.

6 A wide variety of psychoactive drugs are now available for various conditions. These include drugs for anxiety and sleep difficulties, antipsychotic symptom drugs, mood-regulating drugs, as well as others for controlling seizures and hyperactivity in children. Drugs basically provide symptom relief but usually the difficult behavior returns when the person stops taking the drug. Other psychological methods are thus needed along with the use of drug treatment. Drugs have side effects and taken in combination, particularly along with alcohol, may be dangerous.

Prevention and evaluation

Prevention

How widespread is mental disorder?

How many people suffer from mental illness in the general population is a crucial question for mental health programs and preventive efforts. Information about the extent of the particular forms of mental illness which most frequently are found is needed in order to best allocate the scarce resources for treatment and prevention. It is also needed as a base line from which to determine the effect intervention programs have had.

One approach to estimate the amount of mental illness present in a given group is to determine how many people with mental disorders come to practitioners, hospitals, and clinics or are brought to the attention of other settings that keep such records. From these sources we know that in the United States in 1970 there were 20 million people who were diagnosed as neurotic and 3 million as psychotic. There were 5 million diagnosed as psychopathic personalities and 12 million as alcoholic. There were 2 million found to be dependent on dangerous drugs, such as heroin and barbiturates, 6½ million were labeled mentally retarded, and more than 10 million juveniles and adults were arrested in connection with serious crimes.

As large as these numbers are, they represent only those people with emotional disturbances who have come into the existing facilities for help. How many more people with serious emotional problems but who are not in treatment or have not been identified is a question of considerable practical importance. One way of answering it has been through the use of extensive surveys of the population in general.

The classic study of this kind in the United States was a survey carried out in mid-town Manhattan in New York City (Srole and others, 1962). In this study, intensive interviews were conducted with carefully sampled households, residents, and their families. Questions whose answers would reveal key symptoms of mental disorder were asked. Then these responses were judged by psychiatrists as to whether the individual was well or had mild symptom formation, moderate symptom formation, marked symptom formation, or severe symptom formation. The results of this survey indicated that 23.4 percent of the population had a significant level of emotional impairment; however, only 10 percent suffered from an extremely severe impairment. This indicates that almost one in four people in the general population potentially is in need of mental health services. The figures also point to the fact that the extent of the mental disorder is considerable and represents a most serious problem.

A further, more detailed look at the findings of the mid-town Manhattan data confirms what had been found in an earlier survey that the lower the socioeconomic background of the individuals interviewed, the greater the proportion of mental illness found in the group. This relationship was first clearly established by the Hollingshead-Redlich (1958) survey of treated mental illness almost 30 years ago. It has been confirmed in a number of further studies since. These findings point out that the greatest problem—and therefore—the greatest need for help is with the economically poorest people. The findings further suggest that it well may be that conditions of poverty and low social status are very much implicated as factors in the development and the severity of mental illness. In fact, the findings show that not only do the lower socioeconomic people have more mental illness but they also have much more proportionately severe mental illness than do those who have more advantageous life situations.

Age is also a factor associated with the extent of mental illness. Older people, particularly those past middle age and above, as a group have increasingly greater rates of mental illness than do the younger groups. There are, however, no real differences between males and females with regard to the extent of mental illness.

These studies make a strong point that when poverty exists the potential for extensive and very extreme mental illness is greatly increased. It appears that the great stress and frustration of living in poverty situations are the main factors in the greater amount of mental disorder among the poor. Conditions of social disadvantage are associated with poor family support and family breakdown. This is the situation that exists for many of the economically impoverished minority groups. Some examples of this can be noted in comparing the rates of certain disorders for the general United States population and the rates for certain minority groups (Kraus & Buffler, 1979). For instance, the incidence of suicide attempts in the city of Los Angeles in 1970 was 150 per 100,000 individuals. For a group of American Indians on reservations in the Northwest, this rate was almost four times higher, 450 per 100,000. Among rural Alaskan natives (Eskimos and Indians) this rate reached the astronomical figure of 1,450 per 100,000.

Admission rates to state and county mental hospitals for the white population of the United States is 181 per 100,000. However, for the nonwhite population, it is 306 per 100,000, and for the Alaskan natives, it is 341 per 100,000.

Similarly, deaths due to alcoholism, suicide, homicide, as well as accidents, all of which are presumably indications of reactions to mental stress, occur at rates that run anywhere from two to four times higher for native minority groups such as Indians and Eskimos than they do for the United States population as a whole.

These figures are another clear indication that frequency and severity of mental health problems are related to social class level, which in turn is often related to disturbed conditions in the family and social disorganization. Such knowledge about where the most severe problems are is necessary and useful for planning and for delivering mental health services. Such data point to target problems and target populations for intervention and prevention. From it we can know where mental health programs are most needed and for which type of conditions.

Ways to approach prevention

Prevention of mental disorders has been modeled after the same general procedures that have worked well in public health programs to control and eliminate physical diseases. In this method the ways of proceeding against disorders are carried out at three different levels. The first way is to increase an individual's resistance to the disorder by some means. For example, a balanced, adequate nutritious diet provides a healthy body that can resist many disorders. In particular, it provides protection from disorders that result from nutritional or vitamin deficiencies. In mental health the parallels might be to help people resist stress by training them to better solve problems and to cope with pressures. The second way is to reduce contact with whatever it is that causes the disorder. With contagious diseases like tuberculosis or scarlet fever, quarantine or wearing face masks has been used. In mental health the harmful effects of uncaring disorganized families could be avoided by helping to develop warm, loving families and good child-rearing practices.

A third way is to change the environmental conditions under which the cause of the disease develops. An example might be that of removing garbage to reduce the breeding grounds of flies which carry various diseases and by putting screens on the windows and doors to keep the flies out. Changing social conditions that breed mental disorder, such as unemployment and prejudice, would be mental health parallels.

Thus prevention can be thought of as operating at three different levels. *Primary prevention* refers to the methods aimed at eliminating the basic causes of a disorder so that it does not happen in the first place. In terms of mental disorder, a large number of factors have been pointed to as possible causes, but as of now the causal factors have not been clearly identified.

Secondary prevention refers to reducing exposure to the causes of a disorder or otherwise reducing the effect of these causes. This method includes identifying particularly vulnerable groups in the population so that they can be provided with special help early or so that efforts can be made to lessen their exposure to the cause.

Tertiary, or third-order prevention, is the term used in this field for treatment (psychotherapeutic intervention in mental health terms). This level of prevention works to provide rehabilitation for those who have the disorder in order to prevent more severe consequences for individuals who are so afflicted.

Primary prevention

It is obvious that to prevent the basic causes of disorder would be the most desirable means of dealing with it, since when the cause is gone the disorder simply would not develop. In the area of mental illness precise causes of mental disorders are not as yet clearly established. Current evidence points to a conclusion suggesting that there are several or many causes that interact rather than any one factor.

In an approach developed by Gerald Caplan (1970) three factors are considered important in determining whether or not a person will develop in a psychologically healthy manner or be psychologically impaired. First are factors having to do with physical needs such as proper food and nutrition, adequate, safe shelter, safety and protection, and an adequate amount of a variety of sensory input and stimulation.

Next are the factors having to do with emotional and relationship needs. People require social and emotional closeness and interactions with others. Some of the elements of these needs include emotional stimulation and satisfaction, social interchanges, and intellectual challenges. These are the kinds of positive stimulation good families can provide. Prevention measures then need to be directed toward the areas of family and relationships. Finally, there are needs at the level of the culture and society the person lives in. These include the social status of the person, that is, the person's place and role within the social group. This has much to do with the person's sense of belonging, with the person's involvement, and the person's sense of power and importance. All of these factors are crucial in determining positive or negative mental health.

It follows then that people who are living in below-standard housing, or in areas where they can have little sense of protection or security, or in isolation and without adequate stimulation are at very high risk for developing emotional difficulties. The preventive measure for such situations would be to eliminate negative basic factors by providing adequate nutrition, housing, safety and stimulation.

Another social disadvantage occurs when society and culture do not find a useful and important role for some of their members, or when some members are treated as outcasts or treated with prejudice, or are treated as having low status and are not permitted to gain a role or any power. Such disadvantaged individuals are highly vulnerable to emotional difficulties as well. Preventive efforts for those kinds of situations need to be directed toward improving the overall social conditions for these people.

At the level of the individual, helping the person to develop effective ways of coping with life's problems, particularly crisis situations, is most useful. Crisis intervention, as has been noted earlier, is then not just a means of helping a person handle immediate difficulties. It can also be a growth process and a means for handling future problems.

The approaches used for developing programs to deal effectively with these factors are of three main types: (1) those involving major social and cultural areas that can only effectively be dealt with by government programs; a change in basic social conditions is the target; (2) those involving intervention in intimate family relationships and the socializing influences of family, as well as peer groups, and social and religious organizations; (3) those that focus on helping the individual increase his or her capacity to cope with life's problems.

To improve social conditions, what are needed are concentrated basic social action programs such as those aimed at providing adequate nutrition. Examples are the food stamp programs, various school meal programs, and meals for the elderly. Other social action programs would focus on providing subsidized or public housing, increasing the opportunities for jobs, and improving health care. Such things are all largely matters that require governmental action and funding.

One vital social program is to provide medical and nutritional care for pregnant women and for newborn and young children. An equally important need is to provide assistance in the basic skills of being a parent. This includes not only information on proper health care for children but also on the need for proper emotional warmth and stimulation and for encouragement and development of the child's self-esteem.

In this regard, early intervention to provide necessary stimulation for deprived children and to help overcome other handicaps of poverty is important. Examples of effective programs include Head Start and day-care centers for children of working mothers. Other important preventive social measures are the protection of individual rights and the elimination of discrimination and prejudice through equal opportunity. The more positive the atmosphere is, the more the child can develop a sense of worth, belonging, and adequacy.

The role of mental health workers at this social and governmental level of prevention is probably that of providing consultation and information to the legislators and others who have the political power to make the needed changes.

At a more local level, primary preventive work can be carried out most effectively through education about positive mental health and by working toward developing public attitudes that support positive mental health and by working toward developing public attitudes that support positive directions for adjustment. The problems that result from poverty, prejudice, and lower class status are frequently found in the patients of most community agencies. The police, the courts, and the juvenile authorities are most often involved in some of the most severe cases. Providing consultation to these agencies is often most useful, for example, through training and information sessions for police and juvenile workers in order to help them to be much more effective in dealing with family crisis problems.

Another area for preventive work is the school. School is a vital social agency that performs a basic socializing role. After all, since children are in school for a large share of their lives, the school is in a strong position to influence. That school is so involved with children's behavior means that what school does or doesn't do is very important from a preventive mental health point of view. One of the best places to identify difficult emotional problems, difficult family situations, and academic problems is the school. With such information, where to best put preventive intervention efforts can be determined. On the positive side, school can provide positive examples of good mental health and effective problem solving. Through helping children gain skills, confidence, and adequate self-esteem and self-control, school can contribute greatly to the prevention of severe problems later.

Another role of the school is to help children prepare for meaningful and satisfying work in adult life. To the extent that the school successfully does these things, it provides a considerable level of prevention.

Making mental health consultation available to the school, particularly for high-risk children, is a good way to back up the school in these efforts, as is providing information and encouragement to teachers in their work with high-risk children.

It is usually true that people in the lowest social economic levels feel defeated, left out, rejected, and unwanted by the rest of society. Since they often are minority people, they may frequently experience discrimination and prejudice. Very important preventive measures are helping the poor overcome their feelings of helplessness and inadequacy and aiding them to develop the feeling that they can be a part of the mainstream of society and that they can have the power needed so that they can be effective. Assistance to such groups may best be in the form of helping them organize, develop leadership, and learn how to be effective.

From the standpoint of the family, which is the primary basis of relationships and socializing, the important preventive measures can be carried out through programs that work toward helping parents in their role as parents to better understand the emotional needs of their children and to develop increasingly effective skills in parenting. Parents need to be made aware of health and nutrition needs and they need to learn to value and utilize the appropriate health facilities such as those that provide prenatal and obstetrical care and pediatric services. Children need family stimulation and encouragement for schooling and intellectual development. In addition, the many programs for children and adolescents that encourage socializing and group participation, such as Girl Scouts, Boy Scouts, church groups, and YMCA, should be brought into preventive programs and put to effective use.

Probably the most important preventive measure is that of helping each individual learn how to cope successfully with life's problems, stresses, and crises. It is very evident that the more prepared and able a person is to deal with life's problems, the less the probability that he or she will experience extreme or overwhelming disturbance when the stresses and difficulties in life become strong and complex.

It has been well established that there is a definite relationship between emotional disturbance or mental health problems and low socioeconomic status. As has been indicated elsewhere, the lower the socioeconomic level, the greater the frequency of mental disorder in such groups, and further, the more severe are the disorders. Socioeconomic status is also related to a number of other problem areas. Delinquency and crime are much higher in lower socioeconomic groups than in groups that are better off economically and socially. Low socioeconomic status is also associated with children's behavior problems in school and with poor academic achievement. In addition, mild mental retardation is strongly associated with lower socioeconomic conditions.

Thus, there is much evidence to suggest that poverty and near-poverty are very important factors in a great proportion of cases of mental disorder. The implications of this relationship of poverty to emotional disorder is clear. A major approach to primary prevention must be directed toward efforts to eliminate poverty and the poor conditions it breeds.

The importance of the family, especially the behavior and attitudes of parents, is implicated as a major influence in the development of emotional disorder. For instance, studies have shown that children whose parents have been involved in antisocial or criminal behavior are more likely to get into difficulty with the law themselves or drop out of school than are children who come from families that are more conforming and stable. Furthermore, if one or more of the parents has an emotional disorder, there is a highly increased possibility that the children will also be emotionally disturbed.

Battered or abused children are a problem of considerable consequence today. These children are not only likely to develop serious psychological difficulties but the development of their intellectual potential and school performance may also be adversely affected.

There is a substantial body of research that supports the commonsense view that loving, secure relationships and firm directions and expectations are the necessary ingredients for developing well-adjusted children. In contrast, children brought up by rejecting, unloving, and inconsistent parents, or children brought up by parents who overindulge them without providing firmness, direction, and control, will most likely develop social and emotional handicaps in a very mobile society and rapidly changing world. Many new parents in our rapidly shifting and changing society have never learned many of the necessary basic skills required to bring up children so that they will have the best chance to be adjusted and to function well. The skills needed for good parenting can be learned and with them problems of children in families could be greatly reduced which would benefit not only the child and the family but society as well.

Much evidence also suggests that very early experiences and stimulation may be crucial to later development for many basic aspects of personality and patterns of relationships. These factors also appear to include intellectual functioning and academic success, and probably many phases of personality development as well, including vulnerability to later emotional difficulties. The implication is that preventive efforts should be stressed for children in the preschool years.

The influence of schools, for better or worse, on children once they are in the school system has been previously noted. Schools are in a good position to assess various aspects of the health, intellectual, academic, and emotional status of children and to provide needed remedial work or referral. When children do not adequately adjust to school programs and then have bad academic and social experiences in school, they don't learn much and are very susceptible to stress and pressure in their later life. Adolescence is a period of stress for emotionally vulnerable youth. It is a very formative stage of development, and preventive programs are needed that focus on helping adolescents find their own goals and directions, helping them to learn how to comfortably relate to others, as well as helping them to establish increasing independence from their families. Such programs particularly aim to help adolescents develop adequate social and heterosexual relationships, to find vocational direction, and to feel that they belong to society.

Adulthood stages should not be forgotten when planning prevention programs. Each of the main stages of adulthood has phase-specific problems. These include establishing satisfying and productive work directions and establishing close, intimate relationships with others, including those which lead to marriage and children. Accomplishing these tasks well helps the person to feel comfortable and satisfied and to have a good social adjustment. When this is not the case, there is dissatisfaction and that person's potential is wasted. The task of raising families in such a way that children are provided with a sense of security and an opportunity to maximize their development is complex and difficult in our changing, modern world. Skills for adequate parenting need to be learned and properly used in order for the next generation to fully develop emotionally and socially.

There are other difficult adult developmental situations, the stress and difficulties of which preventive measures could reduce. These include career advancement stress and struggle for both men and women who are working, changing of roles and relationships as children leave home, and physical decline and changes such as menopause.

For too many people, retirement and old age often is experienced as a particularly difficult adjustment and vulnerable period. Prevention for the problems of old age really need to start early in life. Such things as developing hobbies, activities, and satisfactions outside work, learning how to use leisure time in satisfying ways, and developing sufficient family and social relationships so as to keep close contact with others when conditions change are a few measures that can be of great help later.

Prevention of physical congenital behavioral disorders

Current evidence suggests that there may be general tendencies present at birth that can result in certain people's being more susceptible to emotional difficulties than are others. The incidence of actually inherited mental disorders is extremely rare. Almost all of the cases that have been found to have much of a genetic or inherited basis involve the most severe levels of mental retardation. Some of these have to do with chromosomal abnormality, such as found in Down's syndrome, or Mongolism, and with certain inherited metabolic disorders that result in brain damage.

There are several emotional disorders that run in families, such as schizophrenia, but the hereditary basis of the occurrence of these has not been clearly established. Therefore, heredity as a major cause of emotional disorders remains a controversial topic. For those few disorders in which a reasonably well-supported hereditary basis is present in either or both parents, there are some tools that can be used for prevention. Genetic counseling methods calculate the genetic risk of having an abnormal child, sometimes quite accurately. Furthermore, in some cases, the actual chromosomes involved are viewed and examined by means of new laboratory methods. Given this information, parents are able to make decisions about abortion or about both temporary and permanent birth control.

Probably almost all mental or physical limitations and disorders present at birth or soon thereafter are the result of a variety of physical factors and not the result of a hereditary factor. As an exmaple, the general health and nutritional status of the mother before she becomes pregnant are important factors in how well she can supply the baby with nourishment during pregnancy. During pregnancy, nutrition and proper diet are of course very important to the development of the unborn child. If the mother has nutritional deficiencies, it may mean that she cannot provide proper nutriments to the child. Consequently, the infant's development, particularly of the very sensitive brain cells, could be affected.

Another factor that can also negatively affect the unborn is disease contracted by the mother while pregnant. It is now well known that if the mother contracts measles, especially during the first three months of pregnancy, there is a high likelihood that the result may be a handicapped or possibly mentally retarded child. Syphilis is another serious disease which the mother can transmit to her unborn child. This can result in severe physical and brain damage even before birth. It has also been found that alcohol drunk by the mother during pregnancy may have a seriously damaging effect on the infant. Heavy smoking by the mother may have a similarly harmful result. In fact, any drug taken by the mother during pregnancy could be potentially too strong for the immature, developing body of the infant and could cause damage. There have even been cases in which infants were born addicted to narcotic drugs because the drugs were passed into the infants' blood from the mothers.

Teen-age and very young mothers are more likely to have children with various physical and mental defects than are women in the more prime childbearing ages of the early to late twenties. Premature birth is much more frequent among teen-age mothers than it is among older mothers, and premature birth is associated with a high rate of childhood disorders.

Thus, the physical health of the mother before pregnancy and during pregnancy, the age of the mother, and the kind of medical care she gets before and during the birth are important factors in preventing disorders before birth.

Secondary prevention

The goal of secondary prevention is to reduce exposure to conditions that cause disorder and to identify the disorder early in order to start treatment very quickly. That way the disorder can be prevented from becoming too severe or from spreading very widely. Identifying emotional disorders and starting treatment early should result in less severe behavioral disorders.

To find out if a disorder is present before the severe symptoms of a disorder are apparent involves wide screening of people in the general or in the suspected population. Screening for emotional disorders is done in several ways. One method is to use paper and pencil screening tests of personality. Another method involves brief evaluation interviews conducted by trained interviewers in the field. Still another method used to identify individuals with warning signs of disorder is to talk with those who have close contact with those individuals. This method might work well with teachers who work with and observe children for a long period of time or with job supervisors.

Secondary prevention measures are most effective when the general public has been given the information and is aware of the early signs of the disorder. Thus, information programs aimed at helping people to recognize their own or others' behaviors that could be a danger signal should be part of a prevention effort. People can be alerted to the fact that behaviors such as greatly increased irritability, difficulty in controlling one's anger, inability to form close and lasting relationships with others, beating one's child or spouse, or feeling out of control are possible symptoms and warning signals of mental disorder that should be further looked into.

Early identification of disorders is not of much benefit unless there are ways of helping the problems. An important aspect of the secondary prevention method is that of providing information about the kinds of help available and about where and how one can receive help. For example, the general public should be informed about crisis-suicide centers and mental health clinics and how to contact them. In addition, public information programs should also work to change people's attitudes and values, which may include very negative views on emotional disorders and mental health treatment. There is still a stigma attached to mental disorder. Providing the public with realistic information about causal factors, such as life stress and how various therapy methods work, is an important step toward getting those in need to come for early treatment.

Service agencies must be prepared to provide early help and give adequate services without delay. There must be no impediments to fast access to treatment. Thus, walk-in clinics and crisis hotlines are very effective methods used in secondary prevention.

Tertiary prevention

Tertiary prevention is concerned with providing treatment for those who already have a disorder. This is really the familiar method of standard treatment programs and procedures. In addition, in recent years there has been a whole wide range of new treatment methods and approaches for those with mental disorders. Only some of them will be mentioned here. The more traditional therapies, including the talking–insight awareness treatments, have been increased and expanded by a variety of new self-awareness methods. *Gestalt therapy* emphasizes the person's being aware of his or her immediate situation and experiencing it as well as acting directly upon it. *Transactional analysis* is concerned with the various levels and states at which a person functions and how individuals interrelate with each other in order to find support and gain from the interaction or become involved in more negative outcomes.

Social learning theories have been discussed in a basic general way in the previous chapter and include a number of behavior modification techniques. These include desensitization, counter-conditioning, reinforcement and punishment methods, and assertive training. A wide variety of *pharmacological* or drug treatments are also available. As noted earlier, these treatments are useful for anxiety, insomnia, and psychotic symptoms and for dealing with mood disorders.

One of the goals of tertiary is to help the person to function again at his or her former level and to help the person maintain his or her role as a productive social individual within the family, on the job, and within the community. Some forms of rehabilitation may require *vocational guidance*, job or school training, and perhaps various therapy methods as well. These often can be started early when the patient is still in the hospital or clinic even when the patient is acutely disturbed.

These measures are continued on an outpatient basis until the patient is once more functioning satisfactorily. There are new programs that allow the patient to be hospitalized only during the day or only during the night. This arrangement allows the individual to spend a substantial portion of his or her life with the family and in the community maintaining social ties.

Self-help organizations for people with mental illness have proved increasingly successful. These groups work through patients who form supporting ties with each other. Recovering patients face many common problems when they leave hospitals or other treatment agencies. It is not unusual for self-help groups to be developed in conjunction with halfway houses. These groups often are organized according to the type of disorder. There are many that handle primarily drug and alcohol problems. Alcoholics Anonymous is a well-known organization that has been effective for many years. There are many others for neurotics, for many kinds of drug abuse, for people who have had severe psychotic breakdowns, and still others that focus on various other related problems and handicaps.

Program evaluation

How effective are programs? This is the crucial question with regard to mental health programs, whether they focus on primary, secondary, or tertiary prevention. Finding the answer is difficult because the problem is so complex. It is certainly not sufficient to go by the impression that a program seems to be doing well or poorly. Systematic and objective evaluation is of greatest importance. It is the basic way to find out if patients in need are receiving effective treatment. Evaluation can also determine whether or not resources are being used in the right places and for the appropriate methods. Being able to demonstrate that what is done works serves as a basis for obtaining the financial support necessary for these programs to continue.

It is a very difficult task to do a program evaluation in ongoing clinics. In fact, they have only rarely been done, and, unfortunately, evaluations have not been done as consistently as an ongoing feedback to a program as would be the ideal.

Bloom (1972) indicates four basic steps in evaluating a program. The first step is to specifically identify the aims or goals of the program. The second step is to clearly specify the population the program is intended for and indicate specifically what problems or disorders are to be focused on. The third step is to indicate precisely the methods and techniques of intervention to be used. And the fourth step is to determine how the information is to be collected. It must be done so that it shows to what degree specified methods were used on those who were treated and to what degree the stated goals of the program were reached. Some other questions that program evaluation needs to answer include: Have there been other changes in the community or population as a result of the program? Is there any indication in the evaluations that some change in methods or goals is needed? What are the costs involved for this program to meet its objectives?

Methods for program evaluation

Putting adequate evaluation procedures into effect in ongoing programs presents many difficulties, which is probably why evaluations are not often attempted. Still the need for them is great. There are several general forms of program evaluation. They differ mainly according to what measure of success is to be accepted for the evaluation.

The most simple and most widely used method is that of *program description*. This form of evaluation essentially presents a more or less detailed description of the program's development and its current operating procedures. The information provided by this method is very limited. It tells something about goals, planning, and day-to-day problems and describes current operations.

Obtaining the *patients' views* with regard to what benefits and experiences they have had with the services of the program is another method. The patients' views are useful because they tell how the program is being seen and experienced by those who use the service. The usual way of obtaining patients' views is to give each patient a questionnaire either following individual treatment sessions or when the treatment ends or even as a follow-up procedure some months or years later. However, it is not always possible to obtain the cooperation of the patients. Some patients may refuse and others may not fill them out. Some may report what they think is expected of them rather than their true feelings. A further difficulty with this method is that it only obtains the patients' feelings of satisfaction. It does not give any clear indication of whether or not patients have changed their behavior or increased their effectiveness.

A widely used method is that of having *outside experts* come in to evaluate a program. In order to do this adequately, the outside experts must first become acquainted with the program, how it operates and keeps records, and then observe the ongoing workings of the program.

When such evaluations are based on a relatively brief time with the program, as is often the case for instance when the experts are available for just a few days, the evaluations may be of some use, but they may also miss crucial aspects of the program. The problem with this method is that the evaluations are based on the experts' impressions rather than on very precise criterion information. Even though the experience of experts may make for greater accuracy than other people's impressions and be more influential, it is still only impressionistic.

A better but probably less practical way of evaluating the effectiveness of a mental health program is to compare the community's known *rate of disorder* for a period of time before the program starts with the rate after the program has been in operation for some set period of time, for example, three years. The effect of a community alcoholism program might be measured by the number of hospital admissions for acute problems associated with alcohol, including such disorders as delirium tremens and alcohol-related diseases, such as cirrhosis of the liver or Korsakoff's psychosis, found prior to the program. Then the number of admissions for the same disorders could be determined at some time after the program had been in operation. If rates had been reduced since the program began operating, this would be an indication of the program's effect. There are a number of other such possible indicators in a community. These include, for instance, rate of mental hospital admissions, suicide rates and hospital admission rates for suicide attempts, arrests for juvenile delinquency, or rates of school dropouts.

Even though these measures are relatively objective and can in some ways make the point with regard to the effectiveness of the program, some cautions are needed and are not free of difficulties. Rates of admission to various institutions may be misleading because they vary according to changing policies. Hence, the change in rates of disorders may not be due to the program. For instance, there may be a period in which mental hospitals have a policy of admitting people with mild alcohol-related difficulties and later change it to admit only those with the most severe alcohol conditions. Here the changes in rates would have more to do with hospital policy than with the effect of a particular preventive program.

A second problem with this approach is that the presence of a program dealing with a specific disorder may, in fact, attract additional attention to the disorder. This in turn might have the result that people who had not before come in for treatment now do when they know about the program. In such a situation, the number of people identified as having the disorder would actually increase, and that would be an indication of the effectiveness of a program, even though the basic aim is to reduce or prevent the difficulty. This was the actual case in several communities when suicide prevention centers were first started. Before the centers opened many people would not seek help or would try to hide their suicidal thoughts and intentions. When the centers were there they felt more free to come for help. But it appeared that with the introduction of the centers there was also a rise in suicide attempts.

Today there still is a general stigma attached to suicide, so it tends to be a very under-reported cause of death. Physicians sometimes try to protect the family by not recording the cause of the death as self-inflicted, especially if there is doubt about whether or not it was suicide. But, as the result of the introduction of these programs, there has been wider acceptance of suicide as a serious problem, and suicide as a cause of death has been reported more accurately.

There is then no one best way to evaluate a clinical mental health service in a community. It can be approached by using various indicators that may provide information on different questions, but all methods are limited. In considering the results of evaluations, it is always very important to know what methods were used in obtaining the information and what the conditions were under which the information was gained. Even if limited evaluations are important and should be built in as part of the ongoing program, it must be recognized that at this stage evaluation of the effectiveness of programs cannot be done very accurately. It can be approached generally, but it cannot provide totally accurate or final answers. Nonetheless, such approaches to evaluation need to be made. Without them there is little or no way to know what effect a program is having or if it is having any effect at all.

summary

1 Knowing how widespread a disorder is is important for prevention efforts. Methods for determining rates of mental disorder in the general population are counting those in treatment facilities, interview–surveys in the general population, and estimates from certain causes of death.

2 Primary prevention aims to eliminate basic causes. Such causal factors for behavioral disorder conditions are basic health and nutrition, adequate shelter, jobs, income, freedom from prejudice, and a sense of social belonging, power and effectiveness, and at the level of the family, a sense of security, emotional support, caring, and belonging. The school can play an important primary prevention role through imparting positive mental health values and skills.

3 Programs to support adults in parenting skills, in vocational satisfaction, and in retirement and recreation are important. Factors of health care, family planning, and genetic counseling need to also be included. Many congenital and later-life emotional behavioral disabilities can be prevented by proper health care.

4 Secondary prevention aims to reduce exposure to causes and identify high-risk cases for early intervention. This can be done through information programs to alert people to early warning signs of emotional disorder and starting interventions early. The school is often a good setting to identify children in the beginning stages of disorders or those of high risk.

5 Tertiary prevention concerns treatment of those who have the disorder. Many new effective treatments and medications have been developed, including day or night hospitalization, self-help groups, crisis treatment, and community–family involvement.

6 Evaluation of the effectiveness of mental health intervention programs is difficult but important. The methods include: program description, which gives information about the goals, development, and current operations; patients' views, in which patients give their impressions of their treatment; outside experts, who assess the programs; and rate of disorder comparison which looks at the number of cases of the disorder present before and after the start of the mental health program.

7 All of these evaluation methods have significant shortcomings, but they do provide a better basis for judging a program's effectiveness than would otherwise be possible.

References

ADAMS, W. J. "Utilizing the Interpersonal Relationship Concept in Marriage Counseling," in *Marital Therapy*, H. L. Silverman, ed. Springfield, Ill.: Charles C Thomas, 1972.

AGUILERA, D. C., MASSECK, J. M., & FARRELL, M. S. *Crisis Intervention: Theory and Methodology*. St. Louis: C. V. Mosby, 1970.

ALBERTI, R. E., & EMMONS, M. Q. *Your Perfect Right*, 2nd ed. San Louis Obispo, Calif.: Impact, 1974.

ALLEY, S., & BLANTON, J. *Paraprofessionals in Mental Health: An Annotated Bibliography from 1966 to 1977*. Berkeley, Calif.: Social Action Research Center, 1978.

AMERICAN PSYCHIATRIC ASSOCIATION. *Diagnostic and Statistical Manual of Mental Disorders*, 3rd ed. Washington, D.C.: American Psychiatric Association, 1980.

BALES, R. F. "Drinking and Intoxication," *Quarterly Journal of Studies on Alcohol*, 6 (1946), 480–99.

BANDURA, A. "Psychotherapy Based Upon Modeling Principles," in *Handbook of Psychotherapy and Behavior Change: An Empirical Analysis*, A. E. Bergin & S. L. Garfield, eds. New York: John Wiley, 1971.

BATESON, G., JACKSON, D., HALEY, J., & WEAKLAND, J. "Toward a Therapy of Schizophrenia," Behavioral Science, 1 (1956), 251–64.

BELLAK, L., & SMALL, L. *Emergency Psychotherapy and Brief Psychotherapy*. New York: Grune & Stratton, 1965.

BIRDWHISTELL, R. L. *Kinesics and Context: Essays on Body Motion Communication*. Philadelphia: University of Pennsylvania Press, 1970.

BLACKHAM, G. J., & SILBERMAN, A. *Modification of Child and Adolescent Behavior*, 2nd ed. Belmont, Calif.: Wadsworth, 1975.

BLOOM, B. L. "Definitional Aspects of the Crisis Concept." *Journal of Consulting Psychology, 27* (1963), 498–502.

――――. "Mental Health Program Evaluation," in *Handbook of Community Mental Health*, S. E. Isolann & C. Eisdorfer, eds. New York: Appleton-Century-Crofts, 1972, Chap. 35.

BOWEN, M. "Family Relationships in Schizophrenia," in *Schizophrenia*, A. H. Auerback, ed. New York: Ronald Press, 1959, pp. 147–78.

CAHALAN, D., CISIN, I. H., & CROSSELY, H. M., *American Drinking Practices: A National Study of Drinking Behavior and Attitude* (monograph no. 6). New Brunswick, N.J.: Rutgers Center for Alcohol Studies, 1969.

CAPLAN, G. *Principles of Preventive Psychiatry*. New York: Basic Books, 1964.

――――. *The Theory and Practice of Mental Health Consultation*. New York: Basic Books, 1970.

COLE, J. A., & RYBACK, R. S. "Pharmacological Therapy," in *Alcoholism: Interdisciplinary Approaches to an Enduring Problem*, R. E. Tarter and A. A. Sugarman, eds. Reading, Mass.: Addison-Wesley, 1976.

DANAHY, S., & KAHN, M. W. "Consistency in Field Dependence in Treated Alcoholics," *International Journal of Addictions*, 1981.

DAVIES, D. L. "Definitional Issues on Alcoholism," in *Alcoholism: Interdisciplinary Approaches to an Enduring Problem*, R. W. Tarter & A. A. Sugarman, eds. Reading, Mass.: Addison-Wesley, 1976.

ELKIN, A. P. *The Australian Aborigines*, 5th ed. Sydney and London: Angus and Robertson Publishers, 1974.

EMRICK, C. "A Review of Psychologically Oriented Treatment of Alcoholism," *Journal of Studies on Alcohol, 36* (1975), 88–108.

ERIKSON, E. H. *Childhood and Society*, 2nd ed. New York: W. W. Norton & Co., Inc., 1963.

FARBEROW, N. L. "Suicide Prevention: A View from the Bridge," *Community Mental Health Journal, 4* (1968), 469–74.

FEHR, D. "Psychotherapy: Interpretation of Individual and Group Methods," in *Alcoholism: Interdisciplinary Approaches to an Enduring Problem*, R. E. Tarter & A. A. Sugarman, eds. Reading, Mass.: Addison-Wesley, 1976.

FRANK, J. *Persuasion and Healing*, rev. ed. Baltimore: Johns Hopkins University Press, 1973.

HOLLINGSHEAD, A. B., & REDLICH, F. C. *Social Class and Mental Illness.* New York: John Wiley, 1958.

HORTON, D. "The Functions of Alcohol in Primitive Societies: A Cross Cultural Study," *Quarterly Journal of Studies on Alcohol,* 4 (1943), 199–320.

IRGENS-JENSEN, O. *Problem Drinking and Personality.* A study based on the Draw-A-Person Test. New Brunswick, N.J.: Rutgers Center of Alcohol Studies, 1971.

JACOBSON, G. F. *"Crisis Theory and Treatment Strategy:* Some Socio-cultural and Psychodynamic Considerations," *Journal of Nervous and Mental Disease,* 141 (1963), 209–18.

JELLINEK, E. M. "Phases in the Drinking History of Alcoholics: Analysis of a Survey Conducted by the Official Organ of Alcoholics Anonymous," *Quarterly Journal of Studies on Alcohol,* 7 (1946), 1–88.

———. "Phases of Alcohol Addiction," in *Society, Culture and Drinking Patterns,* D. Pittman and C. R. Snyder, eds. New York: John Wiley, 1962.

KAHN, R. H., & CANNELL, C. F. *The Dynamics of Interviewing: Theory, Technique and Cases.* New York: John Wiley, 1961.

KAHN, M. W., WILLIAMS, C., GALVEZ, E., LEJERO, L., CONRAD, R., & GOLDSTEIN, G. "The Papago Psychology Service: A Community Mental Health Program on an American Indian Reservation," *American Journal of Community Psychology,* 3 (1975), 81–97.

KELLER, M. "Definition of Alcoholism," *Quarterly Journal of Studies of Alcohol,* 21 (1960), 125–234.

———, & EFRON, V. "The Prevalence of Alcoholism," *Quarterly Journal of Studies on Alcohol,* 16 (1955), 619–44.

KRAUS, R. F., & BUFFLER, P. A. "Sociocultural Stress and the American Native in Alaska: An Analysis of Changing Patterns of Psychiatric Illness and Alcohol Abuse among Alaska Natives," *Culture, Medicine and Psychiatry,* 3 (1979), 111–51.

LERNER, B. *Therapy in the Ghetto.* Baltimore: Johns Hopkins University Press, 1972.

LEWIS, O. "The Culture of Poverty," *Scientific American,* 215 (1966), 19–25.

LIDZ, T. *The Family and Human Adaptation.* New York: International University Press, 1963.

LINDEMANN, E. *"Symptomatology and Management of Acute Grief,"* American Journal of Psychiatry, 101 (1944), 141–48.

MacAndrew, C. "The Differentiation of Male Alcoholic Out-patients from Non-alcoholic Psychiatric Out-patients by Means of the MMPI," *Quarterly Journal of Studies on Alcohol, 26* (1965), 238–46.

Mace, D. R. "Marriage as Relationship-in-Depth: Some Implications for Counseling," in *Marital Therapy,* H. L. Silverman, ed. Springfield, Ill.: Charles C Thomas, 1972.

Masters, W. H., & Johnson, V. E. *Human Sexual Inadequacy.* Boston: Little, Brown, 1970.

McClelland, M., Davis, R., Kalin, R., & Wanner, E., eds. *The Drinking Man.* New York: The Free Press, 1972.

McCord, W., & McCord, J. *Origins of Alcoholism.* Stanford, Calif.: Stanford University Press, 1960.

Parod, H. J., ed. *Crisis Intervention: Selected Readings.* New York: Family Service Association of America, 1965.

Rosenberg, N. "MMPI Alcoholism Scales," *Journal of Clinical Psychology, 28* (1972), 515–22.

Srole, L., Langer, T. S., Michael, S. T., Opler, M. K., & Rennie, T. A. *Mental Health in the Metropolis,* Vol. I. New York: McGraw-Hill, 1962.

Stivers, R. *A Hair on the Dog: Irish Drinking and American Stereotype.* University Park, Pa.: Penn State Press, 1976.

Szasz, T. "Bad Habits Are Not Diseases," *Lancet, 7766* (1972), 83–84.

Tarter, R. E., & Sugerman, A. A., eds. *Alcoholism: Interdisciplinary Approaches to an Enduring Problem.* Reading, Mass.: Addison-Wesley, 1976.

Wagonfeld, M. O., & Robin, S. S. *Paraprofessionals in Human Services.* New York: Human Sciences Press, 1980.

Wiens, A. N. "The Assessment Interview," in *Clinical Method in Psychology,* I. R. Weiner, ed. New York: John Wiley, 1976, Chap. 1.

Wolberg, L. R. *Short-term Psychotherapy.* New York: Grune & Stratton, 1965.

Wolpe, J. *The Practice of Behavior Therapy.* New York: Pergamon, 1969.

INDEX